From Research to Practice in Child and Adolescent Mental Health

IACAPAP BOOK SERIES

The Child in His Family Series (1970–1994)

Vol.	*Year*	*Title*	*Publisher*	*Editors*
1	1970 *1970*	The child in his family *L'enfant dans la famille*	Wiley Masson	E. J. Anthony and C. Koupernik
2	1973 *1974*	The impact of disease and death *L'enfant devant la maladie et la mort*	Wiley	E. J. Anthony and C. Koupernik
3	1974 *1980*	Children at psychiatric risk *L'enfant `a haute risque psychiatrique*	Wiley PUF	E. J. Anthony, C. Chiland, and C. Koupernik
4	1978 *1980*	Vulnerable children *L'enfant vulnerable*	Wiley PUF	E. J. Anthony, C. Chiland, and C. Koupernik
5	1978 *1984*	Children and their parents in a changing world *Parents et enfants dans un monde en changement*	Wiley PUF	E. J. Anthony and C. Chiland
6	1982 *1985*	Preventive child psychiatry in an age of transitions *Prevention en psychiatrie de l'enfant dans un temps de transition*	Wiley PUF	E. J. Anthony and C. Chiland
7	1982 *1985*	Children in turmoil: Tomorrow's parents *Enfants dans la tourmente: Parents de demain*	Wiley PUF	E. J. Anthony and C. Chiland
8	1986 *1992*	Perilous development: Child raising and identity formation under stress *Le developpement en peril*	Wiley PUF	E. J. Anthony and C. Chiland
9	1992 *1990*	New approaches to infant, child, adolescent, and family mental health *Nouvelle approches de la sante mentale de la naissance a l'adolescence pour l'enfant et sa famille*	Yale University Press PUF	C. Chiland and J. G. Young
10	1990 *1990*	Why children reject school: View from seven countries *Le refus de l'ecole: Un apercu transculturel*	Yale University Press PUF	C. Chiland and J. G. Young
11	1994 *1998*	Children and violence *Les enfants et la violence*	Jason Aronson PUF	C. Chiland and J. G. Young

The Leadership Series (1998–2004)

Vol.	*Year*	*Title*	*Publisher*	*Editors*
12	1998	Designing mental health services and systems for children and adolescents: A shrewd investment	Brunner/Mezel	J. G. Young and P. Ferrariww
13	2002	Brain, culture and development	MacMillan	J. G. Young, P. Ferrari, S. Malhotra, S. Tyano, and E. Caffo
14	2002	The infant and the family in the 21st century	Brunner-Routledge	J. Gomes-Pedro, K. Nugent, J. G. Young, and T. B. Brazelton
15	2004	Facilitating pathways: Care, treatment, and prevention in child and adolescent mental health	Springer	H. Remschmidt, M. Belfer, and I. Goodyer

The Working with Children & Adolescents Series (2006–)

Vol.	*Year*	*Title*	*Publisher*	*Editors*
16	2006	Working with children and adolescents: An evidenced-based approach to risk & resilience	Jason Aronson	M. E. Garralda and M. Flament
17	2008	Culture and conflict and child and adolescent mental health	Jason Aronson	M. E. Garralda and J. P. Raynaud
18	2010	Increasing awareness of child and adolescent mental health	Jason Aronson	M. E. Garralda and J. P. Raynaud
19	2012	Brain, mind, and developmental psychopathology in childhood	Jason Aronson	M. E. Garralda and J. P. Raynaud
20	2014	From research to practice in child and adolescent mental health	Rowman & Littlefield	J. P. Raynaud, S. Gau, and M. Hodes

From Research to Practice in Child and Adolescent Mental Health

Edited by Jean-Philippe Raynaud,
Susan Shur-Fen Gau, and Matthew Hodes

ROWMAN & LITTLEFIELD
Lanham • Boulder • New York • Toronto • Plymouth, UK

Published by Rowman & Littlefield
4501 Forbes Boulevard, Suite 200, Lanham, Maryland 20706
www.rowman.com

10 Thornbury Road, Plymouth PL6 7PP, United Kingdom

British Library Cataloguing in Publication Information Available

Library of Congress Cataloging-in-Publication Data

From research to practice in child and adolescent mental health / edited by Jean-Philippe Raynaud, Matthew Hodes, and Susan Shur-Fen Gau.
pages cm. — (IACAPAP book series)
Includes bibliographical references and index.
ISBN 978-1-4422-3171-9 (cloth : alk. paper) — ISBN 978-1-4422-3307-2 (pbk. : alk. paper) — ISBN 978-1-4422-3172-6 (electronic) 1. Child mental health—Cross-cultural studies. 2. Teenagers—Mental health—Cross-cultural studies. 3. Child psychiatry—Cross-cultural studies. 4. Adolescent psychiatry—Cross-cultural studies. I. Raynaud, Jean-Philippe, 1960- editor of compilation. II. Hodes, Matthew, editor of compilation. III. Gau, Susan Shur-Fen, editor of compilation.
RJ499.F795 2014
616.89'140835--dc23

2014004831

∞™ The paper used in this publication meets the minimum requirements of American National Standard for Information Sciences—Permanence of Paper for Printed Library Materials, ANSI/NISO Z39.48-1992.

Printed in the United States of America

Contents

List of Tables, Figures, and Text Boxes

TABLES

FIGURES

TEXT BOXES

Editorial Introduction

Jean-Philippe Raynaud, Susan Shur-Fen Gau, and Matthew Hodes

We are delighted to be able to introduce this monograph which has been produced for the twenty-first congress of the International Association of Child and Adolescent Psychiatry and Allied Professions (IACAPAP) to be held in Durban in 2014. This is the first congress of IACAPAP in Africa, and it takes place at an appropriate time in view of the continent's burgeoning child population, significant economic growth, and wish to improve the populations' health. This monograph has been shaped to reflect the mental health needs of children and adolescents in low- and middle-income countries (LAMIC), including Africa. We also include chapters on topics based on research and practice in high income countries, which may have lessons and implications universally.

The first section of the book takes a child and adolescent mental health services perspective, which encompasses epidemiology, mental health needs, and selected policy issues. The opening chapter by Becker and Kleinman is a succinct summary of key issues in global mental health. The chapter describes the high prevalence of psychiatric disorders and associated burden. Given the low number of health professionals, and especially mental health professionals in LAMIC, the authors propose the involvement of non-specialist professionals and lay people to address the treatment gap. The need for appropriate policies, research, and overcoming of barriers to mental health care are proposed.

Merikangas and He give an account of the key findings from three recent child and adolescent psychiatric studies carried out in the United States. The studies converge in finding a high prevalence of psychiatric disorders, but more severe forms of disorder are found in approximately 10 percent of the child population. It is striking that even in such an affluent and relatively well-resourced society, many youngsters with psychiatric disorders do not access mental health services.

The second section of the book provides summaries of research findings into the mechanisms for problems frequently encountered in child and adolescent psychiatric practice. Maziade and colleagues write on genetic processes in serious child and adolescent psychiatric disorders. They provide a lucid review of the evidence that schizophrenia and mood disorders share several causative mechanisms and that at-risk children exhibit, early in development, many of the brain-functioning anomalies that adult patients display. They go on to show that the known heterogeneity within adult nosological categories may have its origin in conditions occurring across the childhood-adolescence risk trajectory. They propose that different combinations of risk factors or risk endophenotypes should be the focus for researchers and clinical practitioners rather than single traits or anomalies.

Gau and Chiang give an accessible account of the main sleep problems occurring in children and adolescents with psychiatric disorders and epilepsy. They have selected the disorders with high prevalence of sleep problems that may be encountered by practitioners: attention-deficit/hyperactivity disorder, autistic spectrum disorders, epilepsy, and mood and anxiety disorders.The chapter explains the mechanisms for the sleep disturbance by drawing on the recent research findings.

Four chapters of the third section of the book address many of the themes and challenges identified by Becker and Kleinman. Marlow and Tomlinson describe the treatment gap in LAMIC between the need and resources in relation to child and adolescent mental health in particular and describe how professionals with a low level of training, or lay people, may be trained to effectively deliver interventions—"task shifting." The interventions may target child and adolescent mental health problems as well as physical health problems. The following chapter by Klasen and colleagues is highly pertinent to the discussion of task sharing as it provides a systematic review of the effectiveness of interventions for child and adolescent mental health problems in LAMIC. The broad ranging review has identified a surprisingly large number of studies of varied interventions, including individual and group psychological treatments and psychopharmacological approaches for a range of childhood disorders. The review describes the effectiveness of many of the interventions, including some studies that were based on "task sharing," and acknowledges that further studies are warranted in view of the variation in social and cultural context in which they are delivered.

Within the global context, there are sadly many young people caught up in armed conflict. This might occur when they fear or experience attack or persecution and so flee homes and become displaced. In some situations, children are coerced into becoming perpetrators of acts of violence as young soldiers. Betancourt and colleagues have carried out pioneering longitudinal studies in Sierra Leone that describe the psychological consequences of war for young people. They have used studies with sophisticated mixed methods that underpin interventions to improve psychosocial well-being.

In a very different context—Japan—Yokoi and colleagues describe the situation for young people and adults with autistic spectrum disorders. They describe their pioneering initiatives in providing a multi-modal service for young adults with autistic spectrum disorders. They provide data regarding the effectiveness of the service. The need to adapt treatment to the cultural specificity of the patient group and their families is the focus of the chapter by Moro and colleagues. They build on the ethnopsychoanalytic perspective which integrates psychoanalytic understanding with cultural insights. These combined approaches provide understanding of the predicament of the children of immigrants. This understanding also underpins the approach to therapy which involves multicultural teams.

The final chapter by Woollard and Kramer summarizes the evidence base for the efficacy of computer and internet-based programs for the psychological treatment of child and adolescent psychiatric disorders. Many programs exist and they have significant advantages over clinic-based interventions, including their easy accessibility and potential for use by youngsters living far from the clinics. Many programs look as if they hold promise in terms of efficacy, but there may be problems with completion of the programs and benefits for a broader range of youngsters. Nevertheless computer and internet-based programs appear to have great potential, and it can be expected there will be further development, evaluation and use of these applications. There is also interest in the extent to which such programs could be used in LAMIC and so help to reduce the treatment gap.

I

MENTAL HEALTH SERVICES PERSPECTIVES AND EPIDEMIOLOGY

1

Mental Health and the Global Agenda*

Anne E. Becker and Arthur Kleinman

When the World Health Organization (WHO) European Ministerial Conference on Mental Health endorsed the statement, "No health without mental health," in 2005 ("Mental Health: Facing the Challenges," 2005), it spoke to the intrinsic—and indispensable—role of mental health care in health care writ large. Yet mental health has long been treated in ways that reflect the opposite of that sentiment. This historical divide—in practice and in policy—between physical health and mental health has in turn perpetuated large gaps in resources across economic, social, and scientific domains. The upshot is a global tragedy: a legacy of the neglect and marginalization of mental health (Saraceno and Dua, 2009). The scale of the global impact of mental illness is substantial, with mental illness constituting an estimated 7.4 percent of the world's measurable burden of disease (Murray et al., 2012). The lack of access to mental health services of good quality is profound in populations with limited resources, for whom numerous social hazards exacerbate vulnerability to poor health. The human toll of mental disorders is further compounded by collateral adverse effects on health and social well-being, including exposure to stigma and human rights abuses, forestallment of educational and social opportunities, and entry into a pernicious cycle of social disenfranchisement and poverty ("Mental Health and Development," 2010; Patel et al., 2007). Advances in efforts to alleviate the human and social costs of mental disorders have been both too slow and too few.

RECOGNIZING THE MENTAL HEALTH BURDEN

The cumbrous and outsized global dimensions of mental illness remained largely unrecognized until the 1990s, when the population health metric disability-adjusted life years (DALYs), which encompassed both years of life lost from premature death and years lived with disability (YLDs), was introduced. The publication of these population health data in *Global Burden of Disease* (Murray and Lopez, 1996), which was regarded as a public health tour de force at the time, also catalyzed a transformative narrative for global mental health. The DALY rubric, along with standardized diagnostic criteria for mental disorders, allowed comparability across disorders and nations and yielded estimates of the composite burden of mental disorders that were much higher than those recognized previously. In 1995, *World Mental Health* (Desjarlais et al., 1995) outlined an agenda to redress the global crisis in mental health. These and other publications debunked lingering questions about the universality of mental disorders and illuminated the enormous suffering associated with these disorders in low- and middle-income countries, where health care resources devoted to neuropsychiatric illnesses were disproportionately low relative to the corresponding disease burden (Saxena et al., 2007). The scientific discourse, which had been largely theoretical and descriptive in nature, became one that encompassed an applied agenda with translational relevance (Lancet Global Mental Health Group, 2007).

In 2013, further documentation renders an increasingly clear and troubling picture of the enormous global burden imposed by mental disorders. The economic burdens associated with mental disorders exceed those associated with each of four other major categories of noncommunicable disease: diabetes, cardiovascular diseases, chronic respiratory diseases, and cancer (Bloom et al., 2011). Major depressive disorder is the second leading cause of YLDs globally and ranks among the four largest contributors to YLDs in each of the socially diverse regions spanning the six continents assessed in the Global Burden of Disease Study 2010 (Vos et al., 2012). Anxiety disorders, drug-use disorders, alcohol-use disorders, schizophrenia, bipolar disorder, and dysthymia also rank among the twenty conditions contributing the largest global share of YLDs. The aggregate burden of YLDs resulting from mental and behavioral disorders

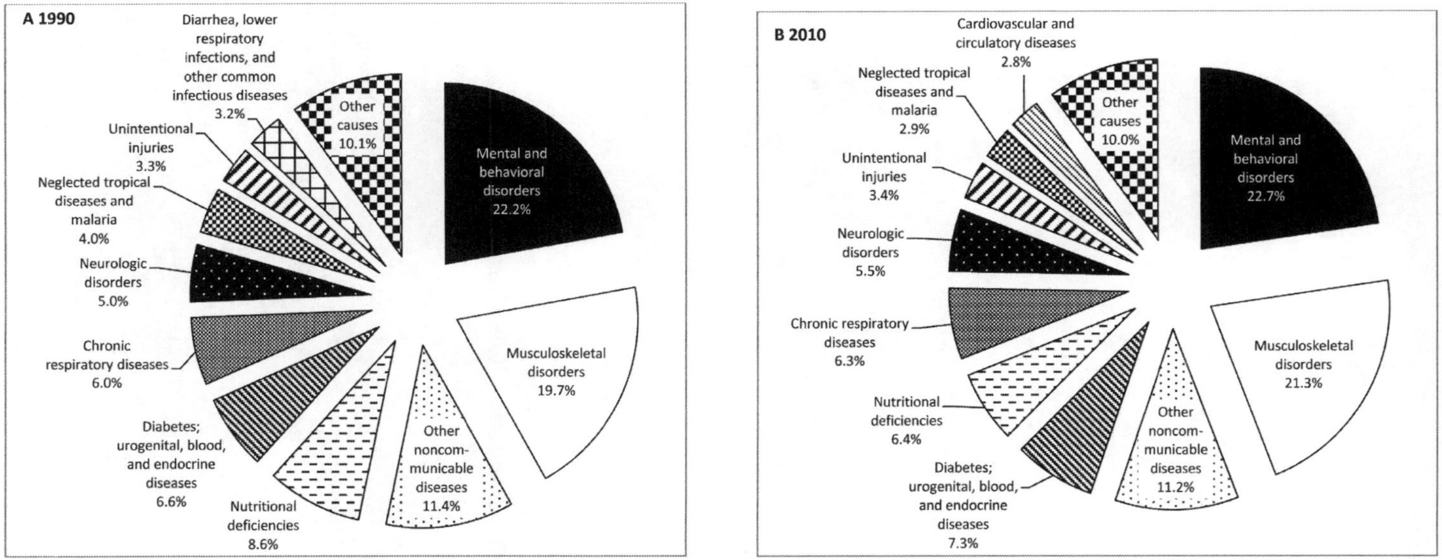

Figure 1.1. **Global burden of years lived with disability, 1990 and 2010. Shown is the global burden of years lived with disability due to mental and behavioral disorders, as compared with disability due to other highest-ranked categories of disorders and conditions. For the year 1990, other causes include cardiovascular and circulatory diseases; transport injuries; neonatal disorders; HIV–AIDS and tuberculosis; other communicable, maternal, neonatal, and nutritional disorders; digestive diseases; cancer; intentional injuries; war and disaster; maternal disorders; and cirrhosis of the liver. For 2010, other causes include diarrhea, lower respiratory infections, and other common infectious diseases; transport injuries; HIV–AIDS and tuberculosis; neonatal disorders; digestive diseases; other communicable, maternal, neonatal, and nutritional disorders; cancer; war and disaster; intentional injuries; maternal disorders; and cirrhosis of the liver. The percentages corresponding to the individual sectors do not sum to 100 percent because of rounding. Categories and data are from Vos et al. (2012).**

(22.7 percent) continues to be higher than that resulting from any other disease category, with an estimated contribution to the proportion of burden in 2010 that was similar to that in 1990 (see figure 1.1; Vos et al., 2012). Yet the game-changing potential of these empirical data to increase global investments in mental health care in proportion to the size of the problem has not been realized. Instead, vast gaps in resources persist and seriously compromise access to care.

CLOSING GAPS IN TREATMENT

More than 75 percent of persons with serious mental illness in less-developed countries do not receive treatment for it (Demyttenaere et al., 2004). For the minority who do have access to mental health treatment in low- and middle-income countries, there are few data available to aid in the evaluation of the quality or effectiveness of the treatment. Major deficits in the provision of care include the size of the health care workforce and the training it receives; rigorous empirical evaluation of innovative, scalable models of care delivery; and the political will to support policy, research, training, and infrastructure as explicit priorities at the national, regional, and multinational levels. None of these deficits can be properly remedied without corresponding advances in the others, creating a Gordian knot familiar to global health advocates and practitioners.

Building Clinical Capacity

The shortage of clinicians with specialized training in assessing and managing the treatment of patients with mental disorders is a major barrier to providing adequate services in low- and middle-income countries (Saraceno and Dua, 2009; Saxena et al., 2007; Kakuma et al., 2011). Building the necessary mental health workforce will require political commitments to elevate mental health to the highest tier of the global health agenda and to develop corresponding national policies that will support the kind of multisectoral planning needed to align educational objectives and resource allocation with local priorities (Bruckner et al., 2011; Celletti et al., 2011). Partnerships among governments, non-governmental organizations, multilateral agencies, and academia can also help to increase the capacity of the mental health workforce ("Scaling Up Nursing," 2009)—for instance, by developing institutional relationships, sometimes referred to as twinning, mirroring, or accompaniment, that would successfully integrate global expertise with local knowledge (Fricchione et al., 2012).

Nonetheless, mere incremental augmentation of the workforce alone is unlikely to close the human resource gap—which is estimated to exceed one million mental health workers in low- and middle-income countries (Kakuma et al., 2011)—given the present capacities to recruit and train mental health professionals (see figure 1.2; Bruckner et al., 2011; "Mental Health Atlas," 2011) and the prevailing models of mental health care delivery. In addition to training more mental health specialists, it is essential to make better use of their expertise by instituting enhancements and innovations that will increase the quality, relevance, and reach of clinical training (Celletti et al., 2011). Resolving the gaps in human resources, for example, will probably entail the use of nonspecialists to deliver mental health interventions (Eaton et al., 2011). This change will call for fresh approaches to training that anticipate the evolution of more prominent supervisory and consultative roles that can leverage the scarce supply of expertise in mental health specialties. The contribution of these specialists must go beyond that of direct service delivery alone. Specialists would be prepared to train and supervise peer nonspecialist professionals to deliver mental health treatment in primary care settings, and nonprofessional health workers would be trained in the tasks of basic case identification, monitoring, and treatment delivery. Novel pedagogic models are called

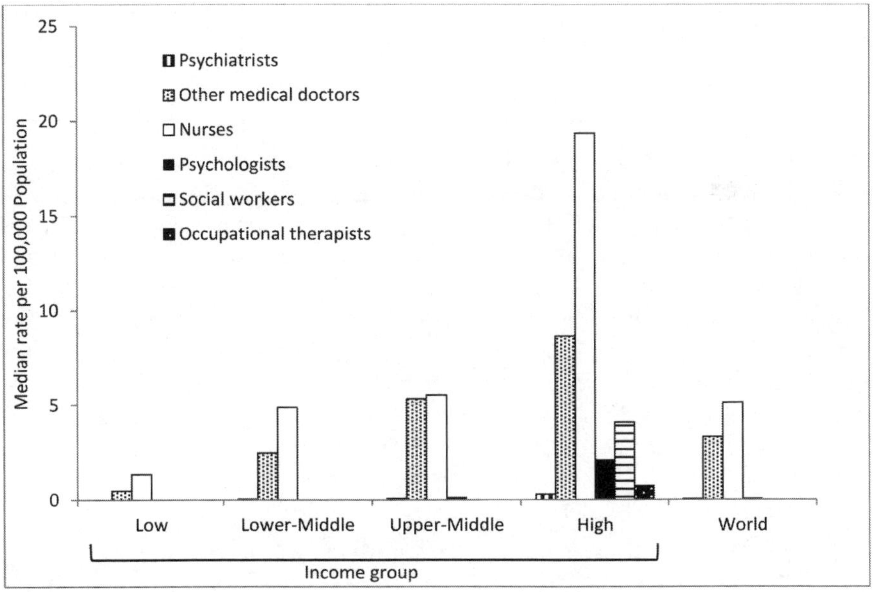

Figure 1.2. Graduation rates among professional mental health specialists in low-, middle-, and high-income countries. Income levels are in accordance with definitions from the World Bank. Data are from the World Health Organization Mental Health Atlas 2011 for the preceding academic year ("Mental Health Atlas" 2011).

for, as are rigorous evaluations of their effectiveness. The implementation of policy that supports the training, deployment, and decentralization of professionals who are qualified for assessing and delivering care for patients with mental illness—and are enabled to do so—will help to achieve meaningful, sustained progress (Saraceno et al., 2007).

Developing New Models of Treatment

The evidence base supporting the efficacy of various treatments for mental health is founded primarily on trials that were conducted in high-income countries. Because only a tiny fraction of published clinical trials have been conducted in low-income countries, the effectiveness of treatments across culturally diverse, low-income settings is largely unknown. In addition, the shortfall of health professionals with training to deliver mental health care in regions with limited resources diminishes the feasibility and relevance of these therapeutic approaches, many of which would require radical adaptation if applied within the constraints of local health care resources. Critics have pointed out that current models that rely on mental health professionals to deliver care to patients are not only unsuitable for low- and middle-income countries (Bruckner et al., 2011) but are also impractical in high-income countries, where adequate numbers of mental health professionals are lacking (Muijen, 2006; Patel, 2009). In this respect, a shift to a collaborative model of care delivery has been proposed. This model reconfigures the role of the mental health specialist collaborative care to emphasize training, supervision, and tertiary care while transferring the bulk of direct service delivery to community health workers or primary care professionals who would receive specific training and supervision in mental health (Patel, 2009).

The success of this model of collaborative care is premised in part on the feasibility and effectiveness of shifting aspects of case identification and delivery of care from mental health professionals to community health workers who receive specialized training, periodic refresher training, and ongoing supervision by professionals. Similar models of "task shifting" in the delivery of health care (e.g., using community health workers in other clinical domains in low-income settings) have been successful, including in populations that are considered to be especially difficult to treat (Behforouz, Farmer, and Mukherjee, 2004; Ivers et al., 2011). Several landmark studies provide conceptual support for this model for the treatment of mental illness in resource-constrained settings, including trials evaluating the effectiveness of interpersonal psychotherapy and cognitive behavioral therapy (Bass et al., 2006; Cohen, 2001; Patel et al., 2011; Petersen et al., 2012; Rahman et al., 2008). These approaches hold undeniable promise for broadening access to effective treatments, but their potential to be scaled up and delivered in a sustained way remains untested and uncertain.

Several milestones mark substantive advances in the integration of mental health care into primary care in resource-constrained settings. Among these are the publication of the World Health Report in 2001 (World Health Report, 2001), which was devoted to mental health; the introduction in 2002 of the Mental Health Global Action Programme (mhGAP), a WHO-led multilateral initiative that encompassed a plan to equip primary care clinicians with training and skills in the care of patients with mental illness ("Mental Health Global Action Programme," 2002) and a series of reviews published in 2009 that provided recommendations on incorporating primary and specialist health professionals as well as trained community health workers into a model of collaborative care that included case identification and management (Patel et al., 2009; Patel and Thornicroft, 2009). In 2010, the mhGAP Intervention Guide aimed to develop clinical capacities in mental health assessment and treatment among nonspecialists ("WHO mhGAP Intervention Guide," 2010). In 2012, the WHO released a training package designed to complement the guide and also encouraged field testing ("WHO mhGAP newsletter," 2012).

These important achievements notwithstanding, there are scant data to allow evaluation of the large-scale feasibility and effectiveness of task shifting or its applicability across diverse settings (Eaton et al., 2011; Patel and Cohen, 2003); the suite of recommendations in mhGAP likewise awaits rigorous empirical evaluation of implementation in low- and middle-income countries that can inform future iterations. Available data are also insufficient to evaluate and refine models for training lay health workers to deliver effective mental health care (Lewin et al., 2005). Serious efforts to incorporate local knowledge, moreover, can ensure that guidance regarding case identification and treatment continues to be refined and adjusted to the structure of a country's health system and the specific needs of its population. The perspectives of cultural psychiatrists, psychiatric epidemiologists, and medical anthropologists on the biosocial complexity of mental disorders and their presentation and course in specific cultural and social contexts will be invaluable in helping to create appropriate approaches to surveillance, diagnostic assessment, and therapeutic innovation. Although some mental health programs are noteworthy for their measure of early success (including those in Kenya: Kiima and Jenkins, 2010; and Egypt: Jenkins et al., 2010), other programs have failed as a result of daunting problems: attrition or reassignment of personnel with mental health training, disinclination to care for the mentally ill, and interruptions in supplies of essential psychotropic medicines (Olugbile et al., 2008; Thara et al., 2008).

Creating a Focused and Relevant Research Agenda

Deficits in the global delivery of mental health services reflect, in part, substantial gaps in scientific knowledge about virtually all aspects of the delivery of such care in resource-poor settings (Razzouk et al., 2010). Scientific publications relevant to global mental health lag behind those in other relatively well-researched and well-funded clinical domains, such as the human immunodeficiency virus–acquired immune deficiency syndrome (HIV/AIDS), malaria, and tuberculosis (see figure 1.3 and the supplementary appendix,[1] available with the full text of the original article at NEJM.org). At the same time, studies of mental health in populations living in regions outside high-income countries are underrepresented in the psychiatric literature (Patel and Kim, 2007), a problem that both perpetuates global health inequities (Horton, 2003; Tyrer, 2005) and entails missed opportunities for important scientific research. A platform for scientific sharing and a research agenda honed to remediate deficits in the delivery of care are urgently required (Tomlinson et al., 2009). Finally, the augmentation of research capacity on mental health in low- and middle-income countries is vital to generating an evidence base that will guide strategic planning and implementation (Thornicroft et al., 2012).

Research is needed to refine diagnostic tools and algorithms for deployment in community and primary care settings, to identify mediators and modifiers of risk and resilience, and to measure the effectiveness of conventional and novel treatment-delivery strategies in a variety of health systems. Implementation and health outcomes research are particularly exigent (Collins et al., 2011). Analyses of the collateral, economic, and social effects of mental disorders may inform policymakers who are interested in understanding the relative cost-effectiveness of various mental health interventions as well as the costs of withholding them. Child and adolescent mental health is a neglected area that is of great concern given the strong evidence that mental disorders are predictors of adverse economic, social, and health outcomes in adulthood (Patel et al., 2007), resulting in costs that are difficult to measure but easy to appreciate. Because adolescents with mental illness typically have difficulty accessing mental health care, interventions that effectively address the formidable barriers confronting them—and other vulnerable sectors of the population—are essential (Thara et al., 2008). Another highly ranked research goal is the integration, to the greatest extent possible, of culturally informed screening for mental illness into primary care services (Collins et al., 2011; Tomlinson et al., 2009).

Overcoming Barriers to Equitable Care

Even in regions in which mental health services are widely available, a sizable proportion of the population with mental illness does not receive

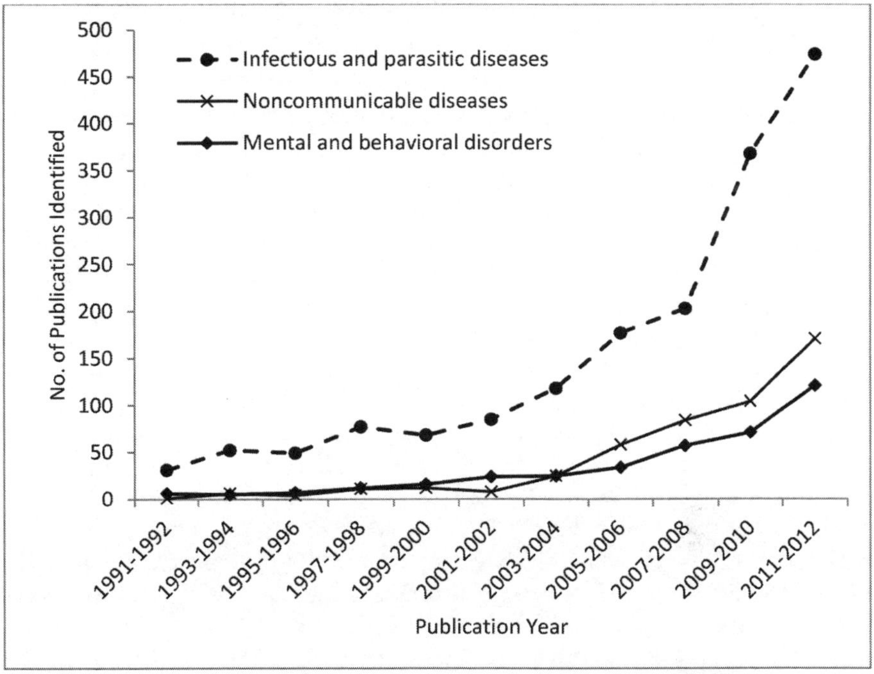

Figure 1.3. Number of scientific publications addressing global or international health, according to broad disease category, 1991–2012. The numbers of publications in the categories of infectious and parasitic diseases, noncommunicable diseases, and mental and behavioral disorders were determined by means of a customized search in the PubMed database for the terms international health, global health, or tropical medicine in combination with one of the three broad disease categories and selected diseases or conditions within them. The latter included terms—and selected common variants or closely related terms—referencing the top five causes of "All ages DALYs" (disability-adjusted life years among persons of all ages) reported for 2010 by Murray et al. within each respective category, excluding birth complications, road injury, and self-harm. The noncommunicable diseases search included the top five categories, excluding mental and behavioral disorders. For more information on search procedures, see the supplementary appendix published online, accompanying the original NEJM publication and available at: http://www.nejm.org/doi/suppl/10.1056/NEJMra1110827/suppl_file/nejmra1110827_appendix.pdf.

care that is specific to the illness ("Mental Health: Facing the Challenges," 2005; Demyttenaere et al., 2004). Cultural practices affect the ways in which people cope with social adversity, manifest emotional distress and mental disorders, and seek care. Economic and social vulnerabilities may make medicines, appointments with health care professionals, and transportation to a clinic unaffordable and time lost from work too costly. For example, even though most low-income countries include psychotropic agents on their list of essential medicines, in 85 percent of those countries these medications are not available at all primary health care facilities. Moreover, the high median cost of psychotropic medicines in these countries is often prohibitive (e.g., the cost of treatment with antipsychotic agents would equal 9 percent of the daily minimum wage, and antidepressants 7 percent) and together with the expenses of other necessary care may impose economically catastrophic costs on patients ("Mental Health Systems," 2009). Social adversity is both a risk factor and an outcome of poor mental health, and it compounds the disenfranchisement that exacerbates social structural barriers to health care.

The most basic cultural and moral barrier to the amelioration of global mental health problems continues to be the enormously negative, destructive, and almost universal stigma that is attached to mental illnesses, to patients with a mental illness and their families, and to mental health caregivers. At its worst, this stigma nullifies personhood and constitutes an abuse of human rights. But other forms of discrimination are more subtle and more structural. Psychiatrists, psychologists, psychiatric nurses, and psychiatric social workers are not the only professionals who are targets of discrimination; it is our experience that health policy experts are also adversely affected by stigma, with the result that many shy away from making mental health care a priority. This situation may at last be undergoing positive change. The Ministry of Health in China has begun to advocate for patients with mental illness and to advance their interests, and similar agencies in other countries have begun to do so as well. There is other evidence that the deeply institutionalized stigma surrounding the field of mental health is being challenged and overcome. This may be the most difficult barrier to quantify and yet the most important to address.

An example of how far we still have to go is the exclusion of the topic of mental health from a recent series of papers, policies, and actions advocating priority for four major noncommunicable diseases on the global health agenda. The very sound rationale for urgent and focused global attention to noncommunicable diseases includes the fact that they contribute to a high burden of disease and to poverty, that they impede economic development and the attainment of other Millennium Development Goals, and that there are evidence-based and cost-effective interventions available to address them (Beaglehole et al., 2011); these same arguments make an equally convincing case for the inclusion of mental health as a priority on the global agenda (Bass et al., 2012; Humayun and Mirza, 2011; Lee, Henderson, and Patel, 2010; Raviola, Becker, and Farmer, 2011).

The collective global investment in the HIV/AIDS pandemic led to the recognition that building clinical capacity, pursuing technological advances, providing training for health professionals and paraprofessionals, and engaging in other means of enhancing the health infrastructure in the service of a particular health intervention have the potential to strengthen health systems and accrue benefits across many clinical domains ("Global Fund Strategic Approach" 2007). The distinct clinical and cultural challenges characterizing mental health care delivery notwithstanding, this sort of investment would also seem to be the preferred direction for mental health.

CONCLUSIONS

According to virtually any metric, grave concern is warranted with regard to the high global burden of mental disorders, the associated intransigent, unmet needs, and the unacceptable toll of human suffering. Compelling arguments have been made that investment in mental health services is a matter of cost-effectiveness, social justice, and even a smart development strategy ("Mental Health and Development," 2010; Lund et al., 2011). Despite the dispiriting near-term forecast regarding improved quality and accessibility of mental health services in poor countries, important advances have been made in the requisite scientific knowledge base and political will to develop and implement policies that can upend these inequities and reset expectations for both the quality of global mental health care and the access to it. Closer alignment with the overarching agenda for global health is evident in the strengthened political commitment to mental health care and in the multilateral partnerships marshaling the resources to improve mental health in countries with limited resources. Several major initiatives have directed funding and attention toward addressing global mental health needs. These include the Mental Health and Poverty Project and the Programme for Improving Mental Health Care, both supported by the Department for International Development in the United Kingdom; the Grand Challenges Canada program; and Grand Challenges in Global Mental Health, led by the National Institute of Mental Health and the Global Alliance for Chronic Disease, in partnership with others. In 2012, the report from the Sixty-fifth World Health Assembly urged member states and the WHO director-general to take bold corrective actions (World Health Assembly, 2012). Mental health has arrived on the global health agenda; establishing it as a priority at the highest level is essential to match aspiration to need.

DISCLOSURE STATEMENT

Disclosure forms provided by the authors for the original article appearing in NEJM are available with the full text of the original article at NEJM.org. Dr. Becker reported receiving payments for editorial work from John

Wiley and Sons, for editorial work, travel, and meeting participation from the Academy for Eating Disorders, and for travel and meeting participation from MA Healthcare, the Succeed Foundation, the American Psychiatric Association, and the National Eating Disorders Association. No other potential conflict of interest relevant to this article was reported.

NOTES

* This chapter is adapted from the *New England Journal of Medicine* (NEJM), Anne E. Becker and Arthur Kleinman, "Mental Health and the Global Agenda," 369, 66–73. Copyright © 2013 Massachusetts Medical Society. http://www.nejm.org/doi/full/10.1056/NEJMra1110827. Reprinted with minor adaptations with permission.

1. Supplementary appendix available at (http://www.nejm.org/doi/suppl/10.1056/NEJMra1110827/suppl_file/nejmra1110827_appendix.pdf).

REFERENCES

Bass, J. K., Bornemann, T. H., Burkey, M., Chehil, S., Chen, L., Copeland, J., et al. A United Nations General Assembly Special Session for mental, neurological, and substance use disorders: The time has come. *PLoS Medicine* 9 (2012): e1001159.

Bass, J., Neugebauer, R., Clougherty, K. F., Verdeli, H., Wickramaratne, P., Ndogoni, L., et al. Group interpersonal psychotherapy for depression in rural Uganda: 6-month outcomes: Randomised controlled trial. *The British Journal of Psychiatry: The Journal of Mental Science* 188 (June 2006):567–73.

Beaglehole, R., Bonita, R., Horton, R., Adams, C., Alleyne, G., Asaria, P., et al. Priority actions for the non-communicable disease crisis. *Lancet* 377 (2011):1438–47.

Behforouz, H. L., Farmer, P. E., & Mukherjee, J. S. From directly observed therapy to accompagnateurs: Enhancing AIDS treatment outcomes in Haiti and in Boston. *Clinical Infectious Diseases: An Official Publication of the Infectious Diseases Society of America* 38 Suppl 5 (2004):S429–36.

Bloom, D. E., Cafiero, E. T., Jané-Llopis, E., Abrahams-Gessel, S., Bloom, L. R., Fathima, S., et al. The global economic burden of non-communicable diseases. Geneva: World Economic Forum, 2011.

Bruckner, T. A., Scheffler, R. M., Shen, G., Yoon, J., Chisholm, D., Morris, J., et al. The mental health workforce gap in low- and middle-income countries: A needs-based approach. *Bulletin of the World Health Organization* 89 (2011):184–94.

Celletti, F., Reynolds, T. A., Wright, A., Stoertz, A., & Dayrit, M. Educating a new generation of doctors to improve the health of populations in low- and middle-income countries. *PLoS Medicine* 8 (2011):e1001108.

Cohen, A. The effectiveness of mental health services in primary care: The view from the developing world. Geneva: World Health Organization, 2001

Collins, P. Y., Patel, V., Joestl, S. S., March, D., Insel, T. R., Daar, A. S., et al. Grand challenges in global mental health. *Nature* 475 (2011):27–30.

Demyttenaere, K., Bruffaerts, R., Posada-Villa, J., Gasquet, I., Kovess, V., Lepine, J. P., et al. Prevalence, severity, and unmet need for treatment of mental disorders in the World Health Organization World Mental Health Surveys. *JAMA : The Journal of the American Medical Association* 291 (2004):2581–90.

Desjarlais, R., Eisenberg, L., Good, B., & Kleinman, A. *World mental health*. Oxford, United Kingdom: Oxford University Press, 1995.

Eaton, J., McCay, L., Semrau, M., Chatterjee, S., Baingana, F., Araya, R., et al. Scale up of services for mental health in low-income and middle-income countries. *Lancet* 378 (2011):1592–603.

Fricchione, G. L., Borba, C. P. C., Alem, A., Shibre, T., Carney, J. R., & Henderson, D. C. Capacity building in global mental health: Professional training. *Harvard Review of Psychiatry* 20 (2012):47–57.

The global fund strategic approach to health systems strengthening: Report from WHO to the Global Fund Secretariat. Geneva: World Health Organization, 2007.

Horton, R. Medical journals: Evidence of bias against the diseases of poverty. *Lancet* 361 (2003):712–13.

Humayun, Q. & Mirza, S. Priority actions for the non-communicable disease crisis. *Lancet* 378 (2011):565.

Ivers, L. C., Jerome, J., Cullen, K. A., Lambert, W., Celletti, F., & Samb, B. Task-shifting in HIV care: A case study of nurse-centered community-based care in rural Haiti. *PloS One* 6 (2011):e19276.

Jenkins, R., Heshmat, A., Loza, N., Siekkonen, I., & Sorour, E. Mental health policy and development in Egypt - integrating mental health into health sector reforms 2001–9. *International Journal of Mental Health Systems* 4 (2010):17.

Kakuma, R., Minas, H., van Ginneken, N., Dal Poz, M. R., Desiraju, K., Morris, J. E., et al. Human resources for mental health care: Current situation and strategies for action. *Lancet* 378 (2011):1654–63.

Kiima, D., & Jenkins, R. Mental health policy in Kenya: An integrated approach to scaling up equitable care for poor populations. *International Journal of Mental Health Systems* 4 (2010):19.

Lancet Global Mental Health Group. Scale up services for global mental health: A call for action. *Lancet* 370 (2007):1241–52.

Lee, P. T., Henderson, M., & Patel, V. A UN summit on global mental health. *Lancet* 376 (2010):516.

Lewin, S. A., Dick, J., Pond, P., Zwarenstein, M., Aja, G., van Wyk, B., et al. Lay health workers in primary and community health care. *The Cochrane Database of Systematic Reviews* (2005):CD004015.

Lund, C., De Silva, M., Plagerson, S., Cooper, S., Chisholm, D., Das, J., et al. Poverty and mental disorders: Breaking the cycle in low-income and middle-income countries. *Lancet* 378 (2011):1502–14.

Mental health and development: Targeting people with mental health conditions as a vulnerable group. Geneva: World Health Organization, 2010.

Mental health atlas. Geneva: World Health Organization, 2011.whqlibdoc.who.int/publications/2011/9799241564359_eng.pdf.

Mental health Global Action Programme: mhGAP. Geneva: World Health Organization, 2002.

Mental health systems in selected low-and middle-income countries: A WHO-AIMS cross-national analysis. Geneva: World Health Organization, 2009.

Mental health: Facing the challenges, building solutions—report from the WHO European ministerial conference. Geneva: World Health Organization, 2005.

Muijen, M. Challenges for psychiatry: Delivering the Mental Health Declaration for Europe. *World Psychiatry: Official Journal of the World Psychiatric Association (WPA)* 5 (2006):113–17.

Murray, C. J. & Lopez, A. D., eds. *The global burden of disease*. Geneva: World Health Organization, 1996.

Murray, C. J., Vos, T., Lozano, R., Naghavi, M., Flaxman, A. D., Michaud, C., et al. Disability-adjusted life years (DALYs) for 291 diseases and injuries in 21 regions, 1990–2010: A systematic analysis for the global burden of disease study 2010. *Lancet* 380 (2012):2197–223.

Olugbile, O., Zachariah, M., Coker, O., Kuyinu, O., & Isichei, B. Provision of mental health services in Nigeria. *Integr Psychiatry* (2008):32–34.

Patel, V. The future of psychiatry in low- and middle-income countries. *Psychological Medicine* 39 (2009):1759–62.

Patel, V., & Cohen, A. Mental health services in primary care in 'developing' countries. *World Psychiatry: Official Journal of the World Psychiatric Association (WPA)* 2 (2003):163–64.

Patel, V., Flisher, A. J., Hetrick, S., & McGorry, P. Mental health of young people: A global public-health challenge. *Lancet* 369 (2007):1302–13.

Patel, V., & Kim, Y-R. Contribution of low- and middle-income countries to research published in leading general psychiatry journals, 2002–2004. *The British Journal of Psychiatry: The Journal of Mental Science* 190 (2007):77–78.

Patel, V., Simon, G., Chowdhary, N., Kaaya, S., & Araya, R. Packages of care for depression in low- and middle-income countries. *PLoS Medicine* 6 (2009):e1000159.

Patel, V., & Thornicroft, G. Packages of care for mental, neurological, and substance use disorders in low- and middle-income countries: PLoS medicine series. *PLoS Medicine* 6 (2009):e1000160.

Patel, V., Weiss, H. A., Chowdhary, N., Naik, S., Pednekar, S., Chatterjee, S., et al. Lay health worker led intervention for depressive and anxiety disorders in India: Impact on clinical and disability outcomes over 12 months. *The British Journal of Psychiatry: The Journal of Mental Science* 199 (2011):459–66.

Petersen, I., Bhana, A., Baillie, K. The feasibility of adapted group-based interpersonal therapy (IPT) for the treatment of depression by community health workers within the context of task shifting in South Africa. *Community Mental Health Journal* 48 (2012):336–41.

Rahman, A., Malik, A., Sikander, S., Roberts, C., & Creed, F. Cognitive behaviour therapy-based intervention by community health workers for mothers with depression and their infants in rural Pakistan: A cluster-randomised controlled trial. *Lancet* 372 (2008):902–909.

Raviola, G., Becker, A. E., & Farmer, P. E. A global scope for global health—including mental health. *Lancet* 378 (2011):1613–15.

Razzouk, D., Sharan, P., Gallo, C., Gureje, O., Lamberte, E. E., de Jesus Mari, J., et al. Scarcity and inequity of mental health research resources in low-and-middle income countries: A global survey. *Health Policy (Amsterdam, Netherlands)* 94 (2010):211–20.

Saraceno, B., & Dua, T. Global mental health: The role of psychiatry. *European Archives of Psychiatry and Clinical Neuroscience* 259 Suppl 2 (2009):S109–17.

Saraceno, B., van Ommeren, M., Batniji, R., Cohen, A., Gureje, O., Mahoney, J., et al. Barriers to improvement of mental health services in low-income and middle-income countries. *Lancet* 370 (2007):1164–74.

Saxena, S., Thornicroft, G., Knapp, M., & Whiteford, H. Resources for mental health: Scarcity, inequity, and inefficiency. *Lancet* 370 (2007):878–89.

Scaling up nursing & medical education: Report on the WHO/PEPFAR planning meeting on scaling up nursing and medical education. Geneva: World Health Organization, 2009.

Thara, R., Padmavati, R., Aynkran, J. R., & John, S. Community mental health in India: A rethink. *International Journal of Mental Health Systems* 2 (2008):11.

Thornicroft, G., Cooper, S., Van Bortel, T., Kakuma, R., & Lund, C. Capacity building in global mental health research. *Harvard Review of Psychiatry* 20 (2012):13–24.

Tomlinson, M., Rudan, I., Saxena, S., Swartz, L., Tsai, A. C., & Patel, V. Setting priorities for global mental health research. *Bulletin of the World Health Organization* 87 (2009):438–46.

Tyrer, P. Combating editorial racism in psychiatric publications. *The British Journal of Psychiatry: The Journal of Mental Science* 186 (2005):1–3.

Vos, T., Flaxman, A. D., Naghavi, M., Lozano, R., Michaud, C., Ezzati, M., et al. Years lived with disability (YLDs) for 1160 sequelae of 289 diseases and injuries 1990–2010: A systematic analysis for the Global Burden of Disease Study 2010. *Lancet* 380 (2012):2163–96.

WHO mhGAP intervention guide for mental, neurological, and substance use disorders in non-specialized health settings. Geneva: World Health Organization, 2010. http://www.who.int/mental_health/publications/mhGAP_intervention_guide/en/index.html.

WHO mhGAP newsletter, June 2012. Geneva: World Health Organization, 2012. http://www.who.int/mental_health/mhgap/en.

World Health Assembly. The global burden of mental disorders and the need for a comprehensive, coordinated response from health and social sectors at the country level. Paper presented at the Sixty-fifth World Health Assembly, Geneva, May 21–26, 2012. http://www.who.int/mental_health/WHA65.4_resolution.pdf.

The world health report 2001—mental health: New understanding, new hope. Geneva: World Health Organization, 2001.

2

Epidemiology of Mental Disorders in Children and Adolescents

Background and U.S. Studies

Kathleen Ries Merikangas and Jianping He

INTRODUCTION

Mental and substance use disorders have now surpassed stroke, diabetes, and HIV as the leading cause of non-fatal illness worldwide, and their impact is growing rapidly (Whiteford et al., 2013). This highlights the increasing importance of shifting attention to the early manifestations, risk factors, and correlates of mental disorders in youth rather than treatment of adults who have already developed these conditions. The aims of this chapter are: (1) to provide a background on the definition and goals of epidemiology and its contributions to our understanding of childhood mental disorders; (2) to summarize the prevalence estimates of specific mental disorders in youth from nationally representative U.S. samples; and (3) to describe key issues and future directions in research on the epidemiology of mental disorders in children.

BACKGROUND: EPIDEMIOLOGY

Definition and Goals

Epidemiology is defined as the study of the distribution and determinants of diseases in human populations. Epidemiologic studies are concerned with the extent and types of illnesses in groups of people and with the factors that influence their distribution. Epidemiologists investigate the interactions that may occur among the host, agent, and environment (the classic epidemiologic triangle) to produce a disease state. The important goal of epidemiologic studies is to identify the *etiology* of a disease in order to prevent or intervene in the progression of the disorder. To achieve this goal, epidemiologic studies generally proceed from studies that specify the prevalence and distribution of a disease within a population by person, place, and time (that is, *descriptive* epidemiology) to more focused studies of the determinants of disease in specific groups (that is, *analytic* epidemiology).

Descriptive epidemiologic studies are important in specifying the rates and distribution of disorders in the general population. The two major estimates of rates in epidemiology are prevalence and incidence. Both are based on the goal of identifying the proportion of cases of a particular index disease in a defined population. Prevalence rates are the number of existing cases in a defined population during a specified time period; incidence rates are the number of *new* cases of a disorder in a defined population during a specified time period of observation (Gordis, 2000). Incidence rates are derived from prospective cohort studies, but they can also be estimated from retrospective cohort studies. Most prevalence estimates in psychiatry include lifetime (the number of cases at any time in the lifetime of respondents, irrespective of whether the disorder is current), twelve month (the number of cases in the population during the past year), and point prevalence (the number of cases at the time of the survey). The most common estimates of prevalence in children are either point or one year because of the lack of reliability of lifetime estimates. Prevalence and incidence rates are generally adjusted for sex and age of the base population.

Epidemiologic studies are also designed to identify risk factors that influence the base rates of diseases in the general population. Differential distribution by sex, age, ethnicity, geographic site, or by exposure to particular risk factors provides clues that may be tested systematically with case-control designs. These studies compare the association between a particular risk factor or disease correlate and the presence or absence of a given disease, after controlling for relevant confounding variables. Case-control studies generally proceed from retrospective designs defined by the presence or absence of a disease in the cases and controls in order to identify potential associations between a particular risk factor or set of risk factors, and prospective cohort studies where the cases and controls are defined by the presence or absence of a putative risk factor, and followed prospectively to examine differential incidence of the disease.

Community study data can also be applied to identify biases that may exist in treated populations and to construct case registries from which persons may serve as probands for analytic epidemiologic studies. Such attention to sampling issues is a major contribution of the epidemiologic approach, as individuals identified in clinical settings often constitute the tip of the iceberg of the disease and may not be representative of the general population of similarly affected individuals with respect to demographic, social, or clinical characteristics.

Application of Epidemiology to Psychiatry

The application of the tools of epidemiology to psychiatry have led to both methodological developments including the introduction of structured and semi-structured diagnostic interviews and statistical methods for estimating prevalence and correlates of mental disorders, and substantive findings regarding the high prevalence of mental disorders in the general population, patterns of comorbidity within and between classes of disorders, sociodemographic and environmental correlates and risk factors for mental disorders, and service patterns in general population samples (Eaton and Merikangas, 2000).

Several recent discussions of adult psychiatric epidemiology conclude that the field has now reached its maturity and that the future generation of psychiatric epidemiology should be used to gain understanding of how multiple risk factors interact over time in producing multiple outcomes (Schwartz and Susser, 2006; Weich and Araya, 2004). It now seems likely that many, or most, mental problems involve a complex mixture of multiple genetic and environmental influences, interacting in a nonlinear and nonadditive fashion.

PREVALENCE AND CORRELATES OF MENTAL DISORDERS IN U.S. YOUTH

Many of the future developments in child psychiatric epidemiology predicted twenty-five years ago by Earls (Earls, 1982) have clearly been fulfilled during the past few decades. A comprehensive review of the field of child psychiatric epidemiology (Costello et al., 2004) noted that the number of observations in community surveys of children and adolescents has risen from 10,000 in studies published between 1980 and 1993 to nearly 40,000 from twenty-one studies published between 1993 and 2002 (Costello, Egger, and Angold, 2005). The results of these studies indicate that about one out of every three to four youths is estimated to meet lifetime criteria for a DSM mental disorder (Costello et al., 2004). However, only a small proportion of these youth actually have sufficiently severe distress or impairment to warrant an intervention (Brauner and Stephens, 2006). Application of the Substance Abuse and Mental Health Services Administration (SAMHSA) definition of Serious Emotional Disorders (SED), a mental health problem that has a drastic impact on a child's ability to function socially, academically, and emotionally (U.S. Department of Health and Human Services, 1999), reveals that about one out of every ten youths is estimated to meet the (SAMHSA) criteria for a Serious Emotional Disturbance (SED) (Brauner and Stephens, 2006; Costello, Egger, and Angold, 2005).

Based on the recommendations of several reviews and advisory panels such as the landmark Surgeon General's report on Mental Health (U.S. Department of Health and Human Services, 1999) and a subgroup of the National Institute of Mental Health (NIMH) National Advisory Mental Health Council (National Institute of Mental Health, 2001), NIMH established several research initiatives to address the lack of national statistics on mental health in children. First, a brief dimensional scale of recent (past six months) symptoms of mental disorders, the Strengths and Difficulties (SDQ) Questionnaire (Goodman et al., 2003), was added to the National Health Interview Survey (NHIS) in 2001–2003. The NHIS assesses close to 50,000 families containing a total of approximately 10,000 youth (ages four to seventeen) each year. Second, selected modules from the NIMH Diagnostic Interview Schedule for Children (DISC) Version 4 (Shaffer et al., 2000) were administered to a sample of 8,449 youth (ages eight to nineteen) in the 1999–2004 National Health and Nutrition Examination Surveys (Centers for Disease Control and Prevention, 2006; Froehlich et al., 2007). Third, NIMH took advantage of the opportunity to collect nationally representative data on adolescent mental health by extending the lower age range of the National Comorbidity Survey Replication (NCS-R) (Kessler and Merikangas, 2004), a nationally representative survey of adult mental disorders that was fielded in 2001–2003. The decision was made to limit the sample to youth ages thirteen to seventeen because pilot studies showed that the interview schedule used in the NCS-R, the WHO Composite International Diagnostic Interview (CIDI) Version 3.0 (Kessler et al., 2009b), had limited validity among youth younger than age thirteen. This NCS-R Adolescent Supplement (NCS-A) was consequently carried out in a nationally representative sample of 10,148 youth in the age range of thirteen to seventeen. The NCS-A was designed to: estimate the lifetime-to-date and current prevalence, age-of-onset distributions, course, and comorbidity of DSM-IV disorders in the child and adolescent years of life among adolescents in the United States; identify risk and protective factors for the onset and persistence of these disorders; describe patterns and correlates of service use for these disorders; and lay the groundwork for subsequent follow-up studies that can be used to identify early expressions of adult mental disorders. In the following section, we summarize the findings from these studies to provide a comprehensive portrait of mental disorders, correlates, and services below.

Studies

National Health Interview Survey (NHIS)

The NHIS is an annual nationally representative sample of adults and youth throughout the United States. In 2001–2003, an Americanized version of the Strengths and Difficulties Questionnaire (Goodman et al., 2000) was administered to the parents of four- to seventeen-year-olds in the 2001–2003 NHIS Survey. The SDQ scoring bands were developed to differentiate low, medium, and high levels of emotional or behavioral difficulties. Children at high risk of serious difficulties were identified by three different scoring methods: (1) high symptom scores, (2) parental perception of definite or severe difficulties, and (3) high symptoms plus impairment. These ratings were validated against service contact or use and other well-established demographic and broader risk factors for child emotional and behavioral problems.

National Health and Nutrition Examination Survey (NHANES) Sample

In 2001–2004, a diagnostic interview was administered to 3,042 children eight to fifteen years old who were evaluated in person at the Mobile Examination Centers (MEC) of the NHANES, a nationally representative probability sample of non-institutionalized U.S. civilians. The NHANES used a complex, stratified, multistage probability cluster design that over-sampled low-income persons, adolescents twelve to nineteen years, persons 60+ years of age, African Americans, and Mexican Americans. The response rates for the youth sample ranged from 79.2 percent to 92.3 percent depending on the disorder or the source of information. There were no significant differences in demographic characteristics between the participants and non-participants. Additional details of the NHANES methodology are available on their website.

Information on mental disorders was derived from the NIMH Diagnostic Interview Schedule for Children, version IV (DISC), a structured diagnostic interview administered by lay interviewers to ascertain diagnostic criteria for the Diagnostic Statistical Manual for Mental Disorders (DSM-IV) mental disorders in children and adolescents (Shaffer et al., 1996; Shaffer et al., 2000; Kessler and Merikangas, 2004). Modules for Generalized Anxiety Disorder (GAD), Panic Disorder, Eating Disorders (Anorexia Nervosa, Bulimia Nervosa) and Major Depressive Disorder/Dysthymic Disorder (MDD/DD) were administered to youth and those for MDD/DD, Eating, Attention Deficit Disorder/Hyperactivity (ADHD), and Conduct Disorder (CD) were administered to the primary caretaker via telephone within four to twenty-eight days after the youth interview. The diagnoses of GAD, Panic Disorder were based on youth-informant alone, ADHD and CD on parent-informant alone, and MDD/DD and Eating Disorders were based on either youth or parent informant. Diagnostic algorithms corresponding to DSM-IV were developed in SAS by the DISC Group at the Division of Child and Adolescent Psychiatry, Columbia University (Lahey et al., 1996).

Four levels of impairment based on six impairment questions were derived for each disorder: Level A = intermediate or severe rating on at least one question; Level B = intermediate or severe level on at least two questions; Level C = a severe rating on at least one question; and Level D = either Level B or C. These questions assessed impairment in six domains including interference with the respondent's own life, family life, social life, peers, teachers, and school performance.

Information on twelve-month mental health service use was collected in each of the DISC diagnostic modules. The question was phrased as: In last year, have you been to see someone at a hospital or a clinic or at their office (for specific symptoms of disorders)?

National Comorbidity Survey Adolescent Supplement (NCS-A) Sample and Procedure

The NCS-A is a nationally representative face-to-face survey of 10,148 adolescents ages thirteen to seventeen years in the continental United States (Merikangas, He, Burstein, et al., 2010). The survey was administered by the professional interview staff of the Institute for Social Research at the University of Michigan. The NCS-A was carried out in a dual-frame sample that included a household sub-sample and a school sub-sample (Kessler et al., 2009a, b). The household sub-sample consisted of 904 adolescent residents of the households that participated in the National Comorbidity Survey Replication (NCS-R), a nationally representative household survey of adults (Kessler et al., 2009a). This sub-sample was interviewed between April 2001 and April 2003. The conditional (on adult participation in the NCS-R) response rate of adolescent respondents in this sub-sample was 86.8 percent. Because the household sample included only a small number of adolescents who were not attending school (n = 25), they were not included in the analysis. The school sub-sample consisted of 9,244 adolescents who were students in a probability sample of schools in the same counties as the NCS-R sample. Schools were stratified by type and selected with probabilities proportional to size. The response rate of adolescents in the sample schools was 82.6 percent. The overall NCS-A adolescent response rate combining the two sub-samples was 82.9 percent. One parent or parent surrogate of each participating adolescent was asked to complete a self-administered questionnaire (SAQ) that contained informant questions about the adolescent's mental health. The overall response rate of completion of the SAQ was 83.3 percent. The full SAQ was completed by 6491 parents and an abbreviated form was completed by 1994 parents, yielding a total of 8,485 parents. An abbreviated version of the SAQ was administered to parents when completion of the full SAQ was not feasible.

Details of the diagnostic and risk factor measures are described by Merikangas et al. (Merikangas et al., 2009). Briefly, adolescents were administered a modified version of the World Health Organization (WHO) Composite International Diagnostic Interview Version 3.0 (CIDI), a fully structured interview administered by trained lay interviewers to generate DSM-IV diagnoses (Kessler and Ustun, 2004). Prevalence estimates were generated for both lifetime and twelve-month disorders. Parents who completed the full SAQ provided diagnostic information about MDD and dysthymic disorder, separation anxiety disorder, ADHD, oppositional defiant disorder (ODD), and CD, whereas those completing the abbreviated SAQ only reported on ADHD. Because prior research indicates that adolescents are the most accurate informants concerning their emotional symptoms, anxiety disorders, mood disorders, substance use disorders, and eating disorders were assessed solely by adolescent report, whereas for behavior problems (ODD and CD) , information from both the parent and adolescent were combined and classified as positive if either informant endorsed the diagnostic criteria for ODD and CD. In the case of ADHD, only parent reports were used based on evidence of low validity of adolescent reports.

Definitions of all psychiatric disorders adhered to DSM-IV criteria. Impairment criteria embedded in DSM-IV required endorsement of some/a lot/extreme levels of impairment or moderate/severe/very severe levels of symptom severity. To more clearly identify disorders that were clinically significant, our definition of severe lifetime disorders used higher thresholds of impairment that required endorsement of a lot or extreme impairment in daily activities, or severe or very severe distress. Severe emotional disorders required both distress and impairment to be present, and severe behavior disorders (ADHD, ODD, and CD) required endorsement of symptom criteria by both the parent and the adolescent.

Findings

Severe Emotional and Behavioral Difficulties

Based on parental report on the Strengths and Difficulties Questionnaire (SDQ), 8.9 percent of youth in the NCS-A had severe difficulties in emotions, concentration, behavior, or getting along with others (He et al. 2013). This was greater than the proportions with severe difficulties reported in the NHIS (4.8 percent in 2003, 5.5 percent in 2002, and 5.2 in 2001), most likely attribution to the broader age range of the latter survey (i.e., four to seventeen years old) (Simpson et al., 2005). The percentage of males with difficulties was almost twice as high as the percentage of females with difficulties in NHIS, while to lesser extend sex difference was observed in NCS-A.

Prevalence of Mental Disorders: NHANES

Table 2.2 presents the twelve-month prevalence rates of mental disorders assessed in the NHANES study. One of eight children eight to fifteen years of age met criteria for at least one of the six DSM-IV defined disorders in the past twelve months prior to the interview (13.1 percent)

Table 2.1. Proportions of youth in the NHIS and NCS-A with serious emotional problems based on the Strengths and Difficulties Questionnaire

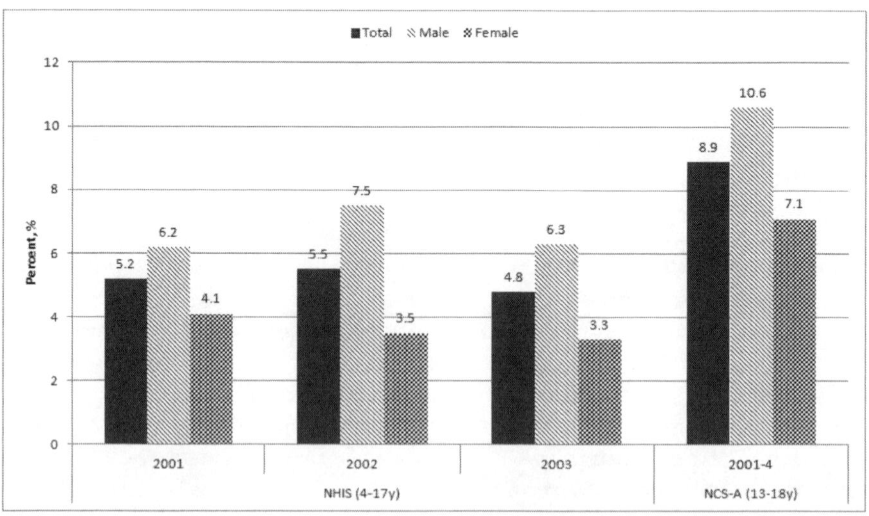

Table 2.2. Prevalence of twelve-month DSM-IV disorders by sex in U.S. children eight to fifteen years of age (NHANES 2001–2004, N=3,042)

	12-month prevalence					
			Sex			
	Total		*Female*		*Male*	
	%	*SE*	%	*SE*	%	*SE*
ADHD	8.6	0.7	5.4	0.6	11.6	1.0
Anxiety (GAD/Panic)	0.7	0.2	0.9	0.3	0.4	0.2
GAD	0.3	0.1	0.4	0.2	0.3	0.2
Panic	0.4	0.1	0.6	0.2	0.2	0.1
Depression (Major depressive disorder of dysthymia)	3.7	0.6	4.9	0.9	2.5	0.7
Conduct	2.1	0.3	1.9	0.5	2.3	0.3
Eating (Anorexia/Bulimia)	0.1	0.1	0.2	0.1	0.1	0.0
Any of above	13.1	0.9	11.6	1.1	14.5	1.0

(Merikangas, He, Brody et al., 2010). Prevalence rates of ADHD were 8.6 percent, depression (MDD/dysthymia), 3.7 percent, conduct disorder, 2.1 percent, anxiety disorders, 0.7 percent (GAD 0.3 percent, panic 0.4 percent), and eating disorder, 0.1 percent. Boys had significantly higher rates of any twelve-month disorder than did girls, primarily because of the high rates of male predominant ADHD. Girls had higher rates of mood disorders.

Prevalence and Patterns of Mental Disorders: NCS-A

Table 2.3 presents the lifetime and twelve-month prevalence rates of DSM-IV mental disorders by sex. Mood disorders affected 14.0 percent of the total sample, corresponding to 11.2 percent who met criteria for MDD or dysthymia and 3.1 percent with bipolar I or II disorder. Females were twice as likely to report mood disorders as compared to males, but the sex ratio for bipolar disorder was more comparable.

Nearly one in four adolescents (26.1 percent) met criteria for an anxiety disorder, with rates for individual disorders ranging from 1.0 percent for GAD to 15.1 percent for specific phobia. All anxiety disorder subtypes were more frequent in females (the greatest sex difference being observed for PTSD). The prevalence of ADHD was 9.5 percent, with more than twice as many males being affected by this condition than females. Any conduct

Table 2.3. Lifetime and twelve-month prevalence of DSM-IV disorders by sex, NCS-A, 13–18 y

	Lifetime						*12-month*					
			Sex						*Sex*			
	Total		*Female*		*Male*		*Total*		*Female*		*Male*	
DSM-IV Disorder	%	*SE*	%	*SE*	%	*SE*	%	*SE*	%	*SE*	%	*SE*
Any mood disorder [1]	**14.0**	**0.6**	**18.1**	**0.9**	**10.1**	**0.8**	**9.9**	**0.4**	**13.6**	**0.7**	**6.4**	**0.5**
Major depressive disorder or dysthymia [1]	11.2	0.5	15.0	0.9	7.5	0.6	7.7	0.4	10.8	0.7	4.7	0.4
Bipolar I or II [1]	3.1	0.3	3.4	0.4	2.8	0.3	2.5	0.2	3.1	0.4	1.9	0.3
Any anxiety disorder [1]	**26.1**	**0.6**	**31.0**	**1.2**	**21.4**	**0.8**	**19.8**	**0.6**	**25.1**	**1.1**	**14.6**	**0.7**
Agoraphobia [1]	2.4	0.2	3.4	0.4	1.4	0.3	1.8	0.2	2.7	0.3	0.9	0.2
Generalized anxiety disorder [1]	1.0	0.1	1.4	0.2	0.6	0.1	0.6	0.1	0.7	0.2	0.4	0.1
Social phobia [1]	5.5	0.4	6.6	0.7	4.5	0.4	4.9	0.4	6.2	0.6	3.7	0.4
Specific phobia [1]	15.1	0.6	16.8	0.8	13.5	0.7	12.1	0.5	14.5	0.8	9.8	0.6
Panic disorder [1]	2.3	0.2	2.7	0.3	2.0	0.3	1.9	0.2	2.4	0.2	1.4	0.3
Post-traumatic stress disorder [1]	4.0	0.3	6.6	0.6	1.6	0.3	3.3	0.3	5.4	0.6	1.2	0.3
Separation anxiety disorder [1]	6.8	0.3	8.0	0.6	5.7	0.4	1.4	0.2	2.1	0.3	0.6	0.1
Attention deficit hyperactivity disorder [2]	**9.5**	**0.6**	**4.8**	**0.5**	**14.0**	**1.1**	**7.2**	**0.5**	**3.7**	**0.5**	**10.5**	**0.9**

Behavior (Conduct or ODD) [2]	**15.5**	**1.0**	**13.4**	**1.1**	**17.6**	**1.4**	**11.8**	**0.9**	**10.0**	**1.0**	**13.4**	**1.1**
Oppositional defiant disorder(ODD) [2]	7.8	0.7	7.3	0.9	8.2	0.9	8.5	0.9	7.2	1.1	9.8	1.1
Conduct disorder [2]	11.2	1.0	9.4	1.2	12.9	1.4	5.7	0.6	5.2	0.8	6.3	0.7
Any substance use disorder [1]	**11.5**	**0.7**	**10.3**	**0.9**	**12.7**	**0.8**	**8.5**	**0.5**	**7.5**	**0.7**	**9.5**	**0.6**
Alcohol abuse/dependence [1]	6.5	0.4	5.8	0.5	7.2	0.6	4.8	0.3	4.2	0.4	5.4	0.5
Drug abuse/dependence [1]	8.9	0.7	8.0	0.8	9.8	0.8	5.7	0.5	5.1	0.6	6.3	0.6
Eating disorders [1]	2.7	0.2	3.8	0.4	1.5	0.3	1.6	0.2	2.4	0.3	0.8	0.3
Any Class [2]	**46.9**	**1.2**	**47.4**	**1.5**	**46.4**	**1.6**	**37.4**	**1.1**	**38.7**	**1.4**	**36.1**	**1.5**
Number of classes of disorders [2]												
1 class	26.6	1.1	26.9	1.4	26.4	1.3	23.0	1.1	23.7	1.6	22.4	1.3
2 classes	11.8	0.9	11.9	1.2	11.8	1.1	9.2	0.8	9.1	1.0	9.4	1.0
3 classes	5.5	0.4	5.1	0.5	5.8	0.6	3.4	0.3	3.5	0.4	3.2	0.5
4-6 classes	2.9	0.4	3.4	0.8	2.4	0.4	1.7	0.4	2.3	0.8	1.2	0.3

Note: Mood, anxiety, eating, and substance use disorder diagnoses are based on adolescent report; ADHD parent reports; ODD and Conduct disorder adolescent and parent reports combined at symptom level using "or" rule.

[1] N = 10,123; [2] n = 6,483

or oppositional defiant disorder was present in 15.5 percent of the sample (7.8 percent for ODD to 11.2 percent for CD), and these disorder subtypes were somewhat more frequent among male adolescents. Substance use disorders were present in 11.5 percent of the sample, corresponding to 8.9 percent of adolescents with drug abuse/dependence and 6.5 percent with alcohol abuse/dependence. These disorders were more frequent in males. 2.7 percent of adolescents had manifested eating disorders at some point in their lifetime, with a twofold increase in rates among females. Finally, 46.9 percent of the total sample was affected by at least one class of disorder, but less than half had disorders with severe impairment (27.6 percent) and only 22 percent exclusive of substance use disorders. The twelve-month rates of disorders were uniformly lower than those of the lifetime disorders. However, the minimal differences in the lifetime and twelve month prevalence rates of ADHD, behavior, and substance use disorders demonstrate the high persistence of these conditions.

Figure 2.1 presents the age-specific incidence curves for each of the major classes of lifetime mental disorder. ADHD was not included in this figure because of the requirement for onset under age seven; thus all cases of ADHD, by definition, would tend to predate those of other disorders. Anxiety disorders occurred earliest with a steep slope beginning in early childhood, and leveling off after age twelve. Risk was fairly low for mood and behavior disorder until early adolescence, when it began to rise steadily. Substance use disorders appeared to have the latest age of onset, with a steep increase in incidence after age fifteen.

Figure 2.2a (female) and figure 2.2b (male) display the proportions of adolescents in the number of major classes of disorders among those affected by at least one disorder. A small majority of affected adolescents (57 percent for both females and males) met criteria for only one class of disorder, most frequently anxiety disorders. Among the disorders from one class only, anxiety disorder is the most frequent condition to occur alone, followed by mood disorders in females, or behavior and substance use disorders in males, eating disorder was the least prevalent disorder to occur alone. About one-quarter of males and females met criteria for two classes of DSM-IV disorders, and 11 percent of females and 13 percent of males had three classes of disorders; and 7 percent of females and 5 percent of males were affected by four to six classes of disorders. These findings demonstrate that despite sex differences in the absolute prevalence rates of these disorders, patterns of comorbidity were quite similar.

Patterns of Service Use for Mental Disorders

Despite the magnitude and serious consequences of mental disorders in youth, only about half of those with mental disorders in the United States

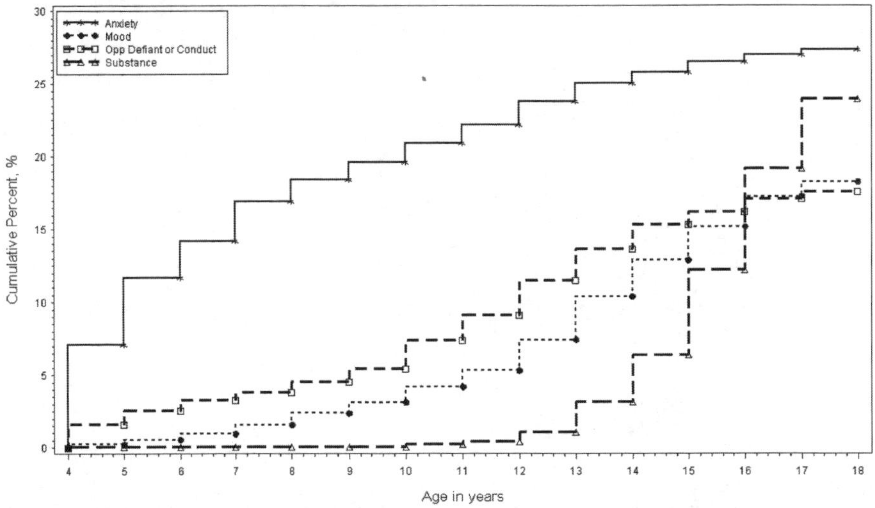

Figure 2.1. Cumulative lifetime prevalence of major classes of DSM-IV disorders among adolescents in NCS-A

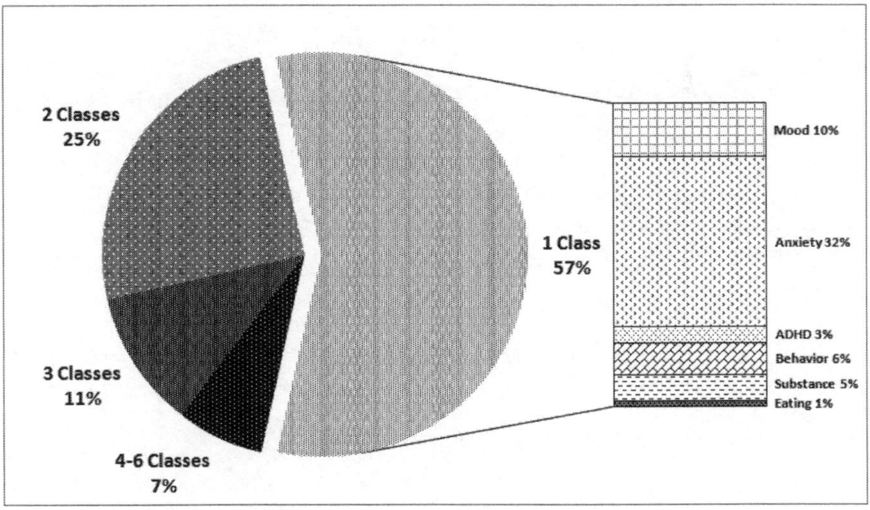

Figure 2.2a. Distribution of the major classes of DSM-IV disorders among female adolescents with at least one disorder (n = 3,333)

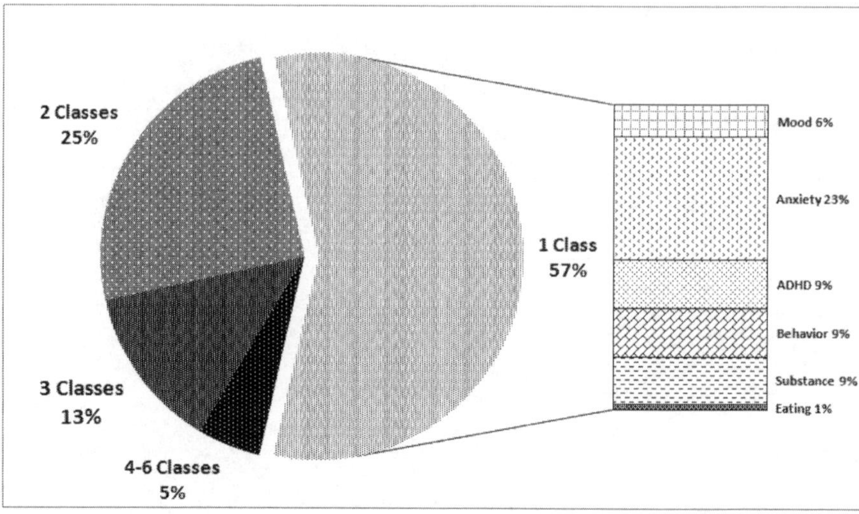

Figure 2.2b. Distribution of the major classes of DSM-IV disorders among male adolescents with at least one disorder (n = 3,150)

receive mental health services (Angold et al., 2002; Canino et al., 2004; Costello, 1988; Kessler and Walters, 1998; Wu et al., 1999). However, a recent review of service rates among those with mental disorders identified in community surveys concluded that those with the most severe disorders do indeed receive service (Ford, 2008). Similar patterns have been reported in the United Kingdom. (Ford, 2008). School services are the most common point of entry for children seeking help, although those who enter through the education sector are unlikely to transition to specialty mental health services (Farmer et al., 2003). The actual diagnostic process and services provided differ dramatically according to the context of entry to service (Hoagwood et al., 2001). A recent comprehensive review of characteristics of youth with service needs in community surveys highlighted the large gap between assessment of mental disorders among those in clinical and community surveys (Ford 2008). Factors associated with service utilization include ethnicity, impairment, comorbidity, suicide attempts, parental recognition, and family burden (Angold et al., 2002; Canino et al., 2004; Fergusson and Horwood, 2001; Lewinsohn, Rohde, and Seeley, 1998; Wittchen, Nelson, and Lachner, 1998).

Figure 2.3 presents the rates of mental health service use for those with each of the mental disorders assessed in the NHANES study. Information on twelve-month mental health service use was collected in each of the diagnostic modules: In the past year, have you been to see someone at a hospital or a clinic or at their office [for specific symptoms of emotional

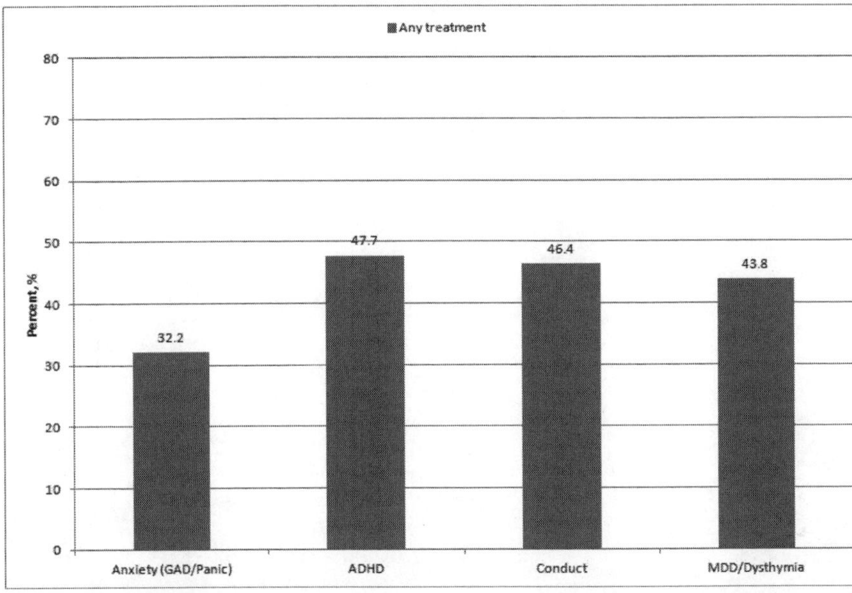

Figure 2.3. Past year mental health service use among children eight to fifteen years of age with twelve-month DSM-IV disorder (NHANES, n = 3,042)

and behavioral disorder?] The results indicate that youths with ADHD and those with conduct disorder had the greatest treatment rates (47.7 percent and 46.4 percent, respectively), whereas those with anxiety disorder had the lowest treatment rate (32.2 percent).

Figure 2.4 shows the proportion of youth in the NCS-A, who received any services for emotional and behavioral disorders in the past twelve months prior to the interview (Merikangas et al., 2011). Service information in the NCS-A was collected immediately following each disorder interview module, in which respondents were asked whether they had received treatment in the past twelve months. In a separate interview module focusing on services, all respondents were asked whether they had received services for emotional and behavioral problems and the settings in which they had received these services.

Of those with any diagnosis, 45 percent reported receiving any treatment from any source. Among individuals with mental disorders, those with ADHD (73.8 percent), CD (73.4 percent), or ODD (71.0 percent) were the most likely to have received any treatment in the past twelve months. Specific phobias (40.7 percent), and anxiety disorders in general (41.4 percent) were the conditions least likely to have received treatment. The rates presented in the figure were based on adolescents and parents reports

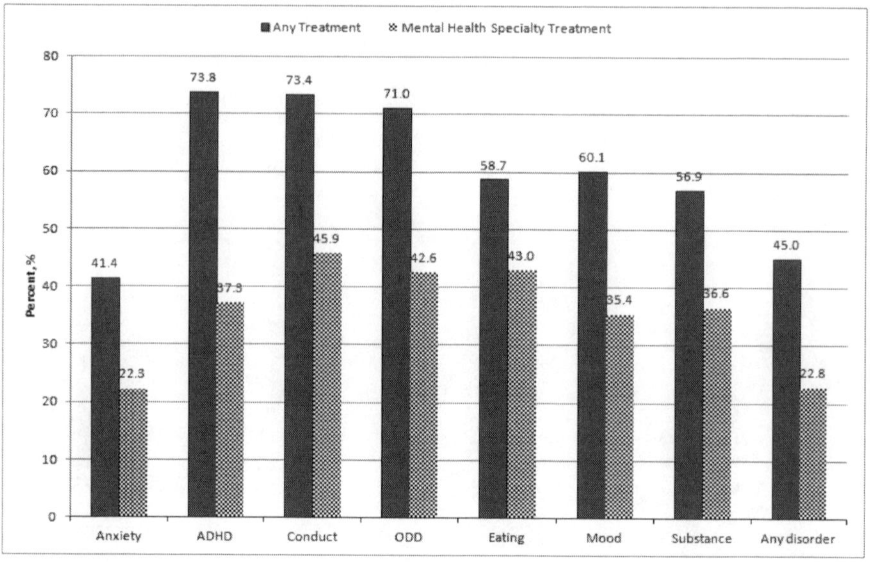

Figure 2.4. Past year service use by twelve-month DSM-IV disorder among adolescents with disorder, NCS-A (13–18 y, n = 6,483).

using "or" rule. Mental health specialty treatment included a psychiatrist or psychologist in settings such as a mental health clinic, community mental health center, drug or alcohol clinic, emergency room service, or admission to psychiatric hospitals and other facilities. Adolescents with any psychiatric disorder were most likely to receive services in school (23.6 percent) and specialty mental health service settings (22.8 percent). Youth with ADHD were somewhat more likely to get treatment from schools (54.5 percent) than from mental health (37.3 percent), while the opposite was true of those with eating disorders (mental health, 43.0 percent, schools 20.9 percent) and drug use disorders (mental health, 44.4 percent, schools, 32.9 percent). The probability of treatment was associated with number of disorders: 68.7 percent of those with three or more disorders received treatment compared with 44.0 percent of those with two disorders, 31.9 percent of those with one, and 14.4 percent of those with no diagnosis. Any treatment included mental health specialty, general medical, school services, juvenile justice, human services, and complementary and alternative medicine. Other details of service use in the NCS-A are presented in Merikangas et al. (Merikangas et al., 2011).

Figure 2.5 presents the prevalence of psychotropic medication use among youth with each of the major classes of DSM-IV disorders. Among those with a DSM-IV disorder, 14.2 percent reported that they had been

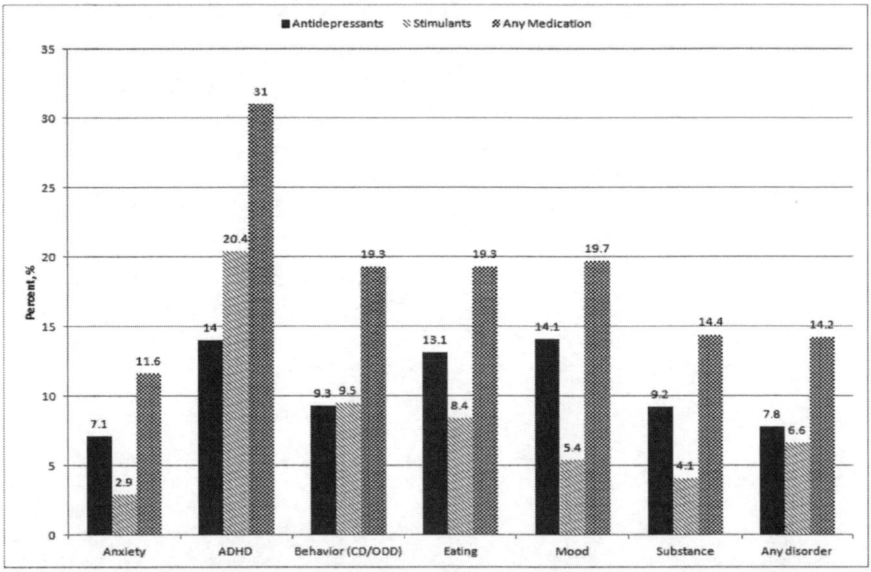

Figure 2.5. Prevalence of psychotropic medication by medication class among those with twelve-month DSM-IV disorder in NCS-A.

treated with a psychotropic medication. Adolescents with ADHD had the highest prevalence of medication use (31.0 percent) followed by those with mood disorders (19.7 percent), eating disorders (19.3 percent), behavior disorders (19.3 percent), substance use disorders (14.4 percent), and anxiety disorders (11.6 percent). Prevalence rates of use of antidepressants (7.8 percent), and stimulants (6.6 percent) were more common than those of use of antipsychotic medications (1.0 percent), mood stabilizers (0.7 percent), and anxiolytics (1.3 percent). (Merikangas et al., 2013)

KEY ISSUES IN CHILD PSYCHIATRIC EPIDEMIOLOGY

Classification of Childhood Mental Disorders

The results of recent epidemiological studies have illustrated the need for further development of the psychiatric diagnostic system (First et al., 2004; Kessler et al., 2006; Kessler and Merikangas, 2004; Kessler et al., 2003; Merikangas, Akiskal et al., 2007). As demonstrated by growing research demonstrating that some diagnostic entities are better characterized on a spectrum (Angst, 2007; Lenox, Gould, and Manji, 2002; Tsuang,

2001), and the pervasive comorbidity between purportedly distinct diagnostic entities, recent studies have begun to expand the diagnostic criteria for mental disorders to collect information on the spectra of expression of particular conditions. For example, expansion of the diagnostic concept of bipolar disorder in the National Comorbidity Survey-Replication (NCS-R) demonstrated the clinical significance of the spectrum concept of bipolarity that had long been described in clinical settings (Akiskal and Benazzi, 2006; Angst, 2007; Merikangas, Akiskal et al., 2007). There is also growing dissatisfaction with the current categorical diagnostic system, which is not believed to provide a valid representation of emotional and behavior problems in youth. Numerous efforts are underway to integrate dimensional and categorical assessments of children (Achenbach, 2005; Hudziak et al., 2007).

Integration of Child and Adult Studies

Epidemiologic studies of adults and children have generally proceeded independently in part because of differences in diagnostic methods and measures, and the requisite inclusion of informant reports regarding child disorders. One manifestation of this independence is the controversy between what constitutes bipolar disorder in adults and children. There has been substantial debate about whether the rapid mood changes and behavioral dysregulation that characterizes children in clinical samples is truly a manifestation of bipolar disorder that has been fairly well-operationalized in adults (Duffy, 2007). There is sparse information on the symptoms of bipolar disorder from community surveys that can address the possible sampling bias in these clinical samples of youth (with the exception of prospective studies such as that of Lewinsohn (Lewinsohn, Klein, and Seeley, 2000)).

The prospective design of many of the community surveys of children and adolescents that began in the 1970s and 1980s has generated substantial information on the continuity of childhood disorders into early adulthood. The cumulative lifetime prevalence of mental disorders derived from these long-term follow-up studies (Cohen et al., 2003; Fergusson and Horwood, 2001; Kim-Cohen et al., 2003; Lewinsohn, Klein, and Seeley, 2000; Reinherz et al., 2003) tend to be even greater than the retrospective estimates of lifetime prevalence reported in adult psychiatric epidemiology (Kessler et al., 2007; Eaton et al., 2007).

Comorbidity of Mental and Physical Disorders

A recent comprehensive review of comorbidity of medical and mental conditions from the Robert Wood Johnson Foundation Synthesis Project

(Druss and Walker, 2011) documented the high prevalence, complex causal connections, and high individual and societal costs of such comorbid disorders in adults using available information (Merikangas, Ames et al., 2007). The bulk of evidence on comorbidity does not include clinical diagnosis of both mental and medical conditions (Gregory et al., 2009), nor do most studies examine a comprehensive range of both of these domains. Moreover, these data have primarily involved adults, and there is a gap in comparable data on children and adolescents in the United States. Despite the call for integration of mental health and medical specialty care in children as reflected in a recent consensus statement from the *American Academy of Pediatrics*, there is a glaring lack of data on the prevalence and course of people with mental and medical disorders in the United States. Although there are data on the prevalence of a range of specific conditions in children such as asthma, allergies, headaches, or events such as injuries or accidents, there is a lack of systematic data on the prevalence of specific medical conditions of childhood and adolescence in the United States. In particular, there is a major gap in knowledge regarding comorbidity of mental and physical health conditions in children who are disproportionately represented in health care settings. Further, while numerous studies employing clinical and population-based samples, as well as samples drawn from systematic databases, have documented associations between a variety of mental health disorders and physical conditions such as asthma (Ortega et al., 2004; McQuaid, Kopel, and Nassau, 2001), allergies (Friedman and Morris, 2006; Slattery, 2005), arthritis (LeBovidge et al., 2003), sickle cell disease (Benton, Ifeagwu, and Smith-Whitley, 2007), epilepsy (Kim, 1991; Rodenburg et al., 2005), and inflammatory bowel disease (Mackner, Sisson, and Crandall, 2004), the majority of prior work that has examined associations between physical and mental health conditions has employed fairly small sample sizes, focused on one or a limited number of physical and/or mental health problems, aggregated many heterogeneous physical conditions together in analyses, and/or failed to control for additional mental health and physical conditions in estimates of association. Finally, most work has relied exclusively on caregiver or self-reports of physical conditions as opposed to employing more objective sources of medical information, calling into question whether observed associations are due in part to a shared method effect or reporting biases (Gregory et al., 2009). Taken together, such methodological characteristics of previous studies greatly limit current understanding of the unique associations between a broad array of mental health disorders and physical conditions among children in general, and disadvantaged children in particular. Nevertheless, this work has generally demonstrated that youth affected with physical conditions are at greater risk for mental health problems relative to youth without such conditions, documenting the need for a more comprehensive data base in the United States (Egger et al., 1999; Lavigne and Faier-Routman, 1992; Bennett, 1994; Cohen et al., 1998; Cadman et al., 1987; Aarons et al., 2008; Boothroyd and Armstrong, 2005; Boyce et al., 2009; Combs-Orme, Heflinger, and Simpkins, 2002; Gortmaker et al., 1990; Hysing et al., 2009; McDougall et al., 2004; Spady et al., 2005; Blackman et al., 2011; Schieve et al., 2009).

SUMMARY AND FUTURE RESEARCH

This chapter provides a comprehensive review of the epidemiology of mental disorders in the United States and its relevance to child psychiatry. There has now been sufficient data in the United States that complements large-scale community surveys in Europe, North America, Australia, and Asia that converges in demonstrating the high magnitude and sociodemographic correlates of mental disorders in children and adolescents. Numerous prospective studies of youth have shown that up to half of youth in the community will develop at least one episode of one of the mental disorders by the time they reach adulthood. However, only about 10 percent to 20 percent of youth meet criteria for a serious emotional disturbance. Although there is substantial variation in the findings based on methodological characteristics of the studies, the findings converge in demonstrating that approximately one fourth of youth experience a mental disorder during the past year, and about one-half across their lifetimes. Anxiety disorders are the most frequent condition in children followed by behavior disorders, then mood disorders and substance use disorders. Variation in the rates across the world can be attributed to both methodological factors and also to true cultural differences in the magnitude of childhood disorders.

However, there is a large gap between the growing evidence base on the magnitude and impact of mental disorders in developed countries and those in developing countries across the world. There is an urgent need to provide resources to facilitate collection of this information in order to develop effective prevention and intervention programs in the parts of the world where the impact of mental disorder is growing. The need for greater integration across psychiatric and medical and primary care settings will also be critical in providing comprehensive portrait of the context of mental disorders and comorbid physical conditions that may lead to greater disability than either condition alone. Finally, there has been a large increase in mental health service uses for children in developed countries that may be attributable both to greater awareness of mental disorders and availability of treatment. However, these patterns are not uniform across the world and greater effort is needed to develop common programs for intervention and prevention that can help to minimize the impact and progression of childhood mental disorders.

REFERENCES

Aarons, G. A., A. R. Monn, L. K. Leslie, A. F. Garland, L. Lugo, R. L. Hough, and S. A. Brown. 2008. Association between mental and physical health problems in high-risk adolescents: a longitudinal study. *J Adolesc Health* 43 (3):260-67. doi: 10.1016/j.jadohealth.2008.01.013S1054-139X(08)00108-0 [pii].

Achenbach, T. M. 2005. Advancing assessment of children and adolescents: Commentary on evidence-based assessment of child and adolescent disorders. *J Clin Child Adolesc Psychol* 34 (3):541–47.

Akiskal, H. S., and F. Benazzi. 2006. The DSM-IV and ICD-10 categories of recurrent [major] depressive and bipolar II disorders: Evidence that they lie on a dimensional spectrum. *Journal of Affective Disorders* 92 (1):45–54.

Angold, A., A. Erkanli, E. M. Farmer, J. A. Fairbank, B. J. Burns, G. Keeler, and E. J. Costello. 2002. Psychiatric disorder, impairment, and service use in rural African American and white youth. *Arch Gen Psychiatry* 59 (10):893–901.

Angst, J. 2007. The bipolar spectrum. *British Journal of Psychiatry* 190:189–191. doi: 10.1192/bjp.bp.106.030957.

Bennett, D. S. 1994. Depression among children with chronic medical problems: A meta-analysis. *J Pediatr Psychol* 19 (2):149–69.

Benton, T. D., J. A. Ifeagwu, and K. Smith-Whitley. 2007. Anxiety and depression in children and adolescents with sickle cell disease. *Curr Psychiatry Rep* 9 (2):114–21.

Blackman, J. A., M. J. Gurka, K. K. Gurka, and M. N. Oliver. 2011. Emotional, developmental and behavioural co-morbidities of children with chronic health conditions. *J Paediatr Child Health* 47 (10):742–47. doi: 10.1111/j.1440-1754.2011.02044.x.

Boothroyd, R. A., and M. I. Armstrong. 2005. Comorbidity and unmet service needs among medicaid-enrolled children with identified disabilities. *Journal of Emotional and Behavioral Disorders* 13 (1):43–51.

Boyce, W. F., D. Davies, S. R. Raman, J. Tynjala, R. Valimaa, M. King, O. Gallupe, and L. Kannas. 2009. Emotional health of Canadian and Finnish students with disabilities or chronic conditions. *Int J Rehabil Res* 32 (2):154–61. doi: 10.1097/MRR.0b013e32831e452e00004356-200906000-00009 [pii].

Brauner, C. B., and C. B. Stephens. 2006. Estimating the prevalence of early childhood serious emotional/behavioral disorders: challenges and recommendations. *Public Health Rep* 121 (3):303–10.

Cadman, D., M. Boyle, P. Szatmari, and D. R. Offord. 1987. Chronic illness, disability, and mental and social well-being: Findings of the Ontario Child Health Study. *Pediatrics* 79 (5):805–13.

Canino, G., P. E. Shrout, M. Rubio-Stipec, H. R. Bird, M. Bravo, R. Ramirez, L. Chavez, M. Alegria, J. J. Bauermeister, A. Hohmann, J. Ribera, P. Garcia, and A.

Martinez-Taboas. 2004. The DSM-IV rates of child and adolescent disorders in Puerto Rico—Prevalence, correlates, service use, and the effects of impairment. *Arch Gen Psychiatry* 61 (1):85–93.

Centers for Disease Control and Prevention. 2007. *National Health and Nutrition Examination Survey Analytic Guidelines* 2006 [cited September 1 2007]. Available from http://www.cdc.gov/nchs/about/major/nhanes/nhanes2003-2004/analytical_guidelines.htm.

Cohen, P., S. Kasen, H. Chen, C. Hartmark, and K. Gordon. 2003. Variations in patterns of developmental transitions in the emerging adulthood period. *Dev Psychol* 39 (4):657–69.

Cohen, P., D. S. Pine, A. Must, S. Kasen, and J. Brook. 1998. Prospective associations between somatic illness and mental illness from childhood to adulthood. *Am J Epidemiol* 147 (3):232–39.

Combs-Orme, T., C. A. Heflinger, and C. G. Simpkins. 2002. Comorbidity of mental health problems and chronic health conditions in children. *Journal of Emotional and Behavioral Disorders* 10 (2):116–125.

Costello, E. J. 1988. Primary care, pediatric and child psycho-pathology: A review. *Pediatrics*.

Costello, E. J., H. Egger, and A. Angold. 2005. 10-year research update review: The epidemiology of child and adolescent psychiatric disorders: I. Methods and public health burden. *Journal of the American Academy of Child and Adolescent Psychiatry* 44 (10):972–86.

Costello, E. J., S. Mustillo, G. Keller, and A. Angold. 2004. Prevalence of psychiatric disorders in childhood and adolescence. In *Mental Health Services: A Public Health Perspective, Second Edition*, edited by B. L. Levin, J. Petrila, and K. D. Hennessy, 111–128. Oxford: Oxford University Press.

Druss, B. G., and E. R. Walker. 2011. Mental disorders and medical comorbidity. *Synth Proj Res Synth Rep* (21):1–26.

Duffy, A. 2007. Does bipolar disorder exist in children? A selected review. *Canadian Journal of Psychiatry-Revue Canadienne De Psychiatrie* 52 (7):409–17.

Earls, F. 1982. Epidemiology and child psychiatry: future prospects. *Compr Psychiatry* 23 (1):75–84.

Eaton, W. W., A. Kalaydjian, D. O. Scharfstein, B. Mezuk, and Y. Ding. 2007. Prevalence and incidence of depressive disorder: The Baltimore ECA follow-up, 1981–2004. *Acta Psychiatrica Scandinavica* 116 (3):182–88.

Eaton, W. W., and K. R. Merikangas. 2000. Psychiatric epidemiology: Progress and prospects in the year 2000. *Epidemiol Rev* 22 (1):29–34.

Egger, H. L., E. J. Costello, A. Erkanli, and A. Angold. 1999. Somatic complaints and psychopathology in children and adolescents: Stomach aches, musculoskeletal pains, and headaches. *J Am Acad Child Adolesc Psychiatry* 38 (7):852–60. doi: S0890-8567(09)66534-5 [pii] 10.1097/00004583-199907000-00015.

Farmer, E. M., B. J. Burns, S. D. Phillips, A. Angold, and E. J. Costello. 2003. Pathways into and through mental health services for children and adolescents. *Psychiatr Serv* 54 (1):60–66.

Fergusson, D. M., and L. J. Horwood. 2001. The Christchurch Health and Development Study: Review of findings on child and adolescent mental health. *Aust N Z J Psychiatry* 35 (3):287–96.

First, M. B., H. A. Pincus, J. B. Levine, J. B. Williams, B. Ustun, and R. Peele. 2004. Clinical utility as a criterion for revising psychiatric diagnoses. *Am J Psychiatry* 161 (6):946–54.

Ford, T. 2008. Practitioner review: How can epidemiology help us plan and deliver effective child and adolescent mental health services? *J Child Psychol Psychiatry* 49 (9):900–14.

Ford, T., R. Goodman, and H. Meltzer. 2003. The British child and adolescent mental health survey 1999: The prevalence of DSM-IV disorders. *Journal of the American Academy of Child and Adolescent Psychiatry* 42 (10):1203–1211. doi: 10.1097/01.chi.0000081820.25107.ae.

Friedman, A. H., and T. L. Morris. 2006. Allergies and anxiety in children and adolescents: A review of the literature. *Journal of Clinical Psychology in Medical Settings* 13 (3):323–335.

Froehlich, T. E., B. P. Lanphear, J. N. Epstein, W. J. Barbaresi, S. K. Katusic, and R. S. Kahn. 2007. Prevalence, recognition, and treatment of attention-deficit/hyperactivity disorder in a national sample of US children. *Arch Pediatr Adolesc Med* 161 (9):857–64.

Goodman, R., T. Ford, H. Simmons, R. Gatward, and H. Meltzer. 2000. Using the Strengths and Difficulties Questionnaire (SDQ) to screen for child psychiatric disorders in a community sample. *Br J Psychiatry* 177:534–39.

Goodman, R., T. Ford, H. Simmons, R. Gatward, and H. Meltzer. 2003. Using the Strengths and Difficulties Questionnaire (SDQ) to screen for child psychiatric disorders in a community sample. *Int Rev Psychiatry* 15 (1-2):166–72.

Gordis, E. 2000. Contributions of behavioral science to alcohol research: Understanding who is at risk and why. *Exp Clin Psychopharmacol* 8 (3):264–70.

Gortmaker, S. L., D. K. Walker, M. Weitzman, and A. M. Sobol. 1990. Chronic conditions, socioeconomic risks, and behavioral problems in children and adolescents. *Pediatrics* 85 (3):267–76.

Gregory, A. M., A. Caspi, T. E. Moffitt, B. J. Milne, R. Poulton, and M. R. Sears. 2009. Links between anxiety and allergies: Psychobiological reality or possible methodological bias. *Journal of Personality* 77 (2):347–362.

He, J. P., M. Burstein, A. Schmitz, and K. R. Merikangas. 2013. The Strengths and Difficulties Questionnaire (SDQ): The factor structure and scale validation in U.S adolescents. *J Abnorm Child Psychol* 41 (4):583–95. doi: 10.1007/s10802-012-9696-6.

Hoagwood, K., B. J. Burns, L. Kiser, H. Ringeisen, and S. K. Schoenwald. 2001. Evidence-based practice in child and adolescent mental health services. *Psychiatric Services* 52 (9):1179–89.

Hudziak, J. J., T. M. Achenbach, R. R. Althoff, and D. S. Pine. 2007. A dimensional approach to developmental psychopathology. *Int J Methods Psychiatr Res* 16 Suppl 1 2007:S16–23.

Hysing, M., I. Elgen, C. Gillberg, and A. J. Lundervold. 2009. Emotional and behavioural problems in subgroups of children with chronic illness: Results from a large-scale population study. *Child Care Health Dev* 35 (4):527–33. doi: 10.1111/j.1365-2214.2009.00967.x CCH967 [pii].

Kessler, R. C., H. S. Akiskal, J. Angst, M. Guyer, R. M. Hirschfeld, K. R. Merikangas, and P. E. Stang. 2006. Validity of the assessment of bipolar spectrum disorders in the WHO CIDI 3.0. *Journal of Affective Disorders* 96 (3):259–69.

Kessler, R. C., G. P. Amminger, S. Aguilar-Gaxiola, J. Alonso, S. Lee, and T. B. Ustun. 2007. Age of onset of mental disorders: a review of recent literature. *Curr Opin Psychiatry* 20 (4):359–64.

Kessler, R. C., S. Avenevoli, E. J. Costello, J. G. Green, M. J. Gruber, S. Heeringa, K. R. Merikangas, B. E. Pennell, N. A. Sampson, and A. M. Zaslavsky. 2009a. Design and field procedures in the US National Comorbidity Survey Replication Adolescent Supplement (NCS-A). *Int J Methods Psychiatr Res* 18 (2):69–83. doi: 10.1002/mpr.279.

Kessler, R. C., S. Avenevoli, E. J. Costello, J. G. Green, M. J. Gruber, S. Heeringa, K. R. Merikangas, B. E. Pennell, N. A. Sampson, and A. M. Zaslavsky. 2009b. National comorbidity survey replication adolescent supplement (NCS-A): II. Overview and design. *J Am Acad Child Adolesc Psychiatry* 48 (4):380–85. doi: 10.1097/CHI.0b013e3181999705.

Kessler, R. C., and K. R. Merikangas. 2004. The National Comorbidity Survey Replication (NCS-R): Background and aims. *Int J Methods Psychiatr Res* 13 (2):60–68.

Kessler, R. C., K. R. Merikangas, P. Berglund, W. W. Eaton, D. S. Koretz, and E. E. Walters. 2003. Mild disorders should not be eliminated from the DSM-V. *Arch Gen Psychiatry* 60 (11):1117–22.

Kessler, R. C., and T. B. Ustun. 2004. The World Mental Health (WMH) survey initiative version of the World Health Organization (WHO) Composite International Diagnostic Interview (CIDI). *Int J Methods Psychiatr Res* 13 (2):93–121.

Kessler, R. C., and E. E. Walters. 1998. Epidemiology of DSM-III-R major depression and minor depression among adolescents and young adults in the National Comorbidity Survey. *Depress Anxiety* 7 (1):3–14.

Kim-Cohen, J., A. Caspi, T. E. Moffitt, H. Harrington, B. J. Milne, and R. Poulton. 2003. Prior juvenile diagnoses in adults with mental disorder: Developmental follow-back of a prospective-longitudinal cohort. *Arch Gen Psychiatry* 60 (7):709–17.

Kim, W. J. 1991. Psychiatric aspects of epileptic children and adolescents. *J Am Acad Child Adolesc Psychiatry* 30 (6):874–86. doi: S0890-8567(09)64359-8 [pii] 10.1097/00004583-199111000-00003.

Lahey, B. B., E. W. Flagg, H. R. Bird, M. E. Schwab-Stone, G. Canino, M. K. Dulcan, P. J. Leaf, M. Davies, D. Brogan, K. Bourdon, S. M. Horwitz, M. Rubio-Stipec, D. H. Freeman, J. H. Lichtman, D. Shaffer, S. H. Goodman, W. E. Narrow, M. M. Weissman, D. B. Kandel, P. S. Jensen, J. E. Richters, and D. A. Regier. 1996. The NIMH Methods for the Epidemiology of Child and Adolescent Mental Disorders (MECA) Study: Background and methodology. *J Am Acad Child Adolesc Psychiatry* 35 (7):855–64.

Lavigne, J. V., and J. Faier-Routman. 1992. Psychological adjustment to pediatric physical disorders: A meta-analytic review. *J Pediatr Psychol* 17 (2):133–57.

LeBovidge, J. S., J. V. Lavigne, G. R. Donenberg, and M. L. Miller. 2003. Psychological adjustment of children and adolescents with chronic arthritis: A meta-analytic review. *J Pediatr Psychol* 28 (1):29–39.

Lenox, R. H., T. D. Gould, and H. K. Manji. 2002. Endophenotypes in bipolar disorder. *Am J Med Genet* 114 (4):391–406.

Lewinsohn, P. M., D. N. Klein, and J. R. Seeley. 2000. Bipolar disorder during adolescence and young adulthood in a community sample. *Bipolar Disorders* 2 (3):281–293.

Lewinsohn, P. M., P. Rohde, and J. R. Seeley. 1998. Major depressive disorder in older adolescents: Prevalence, risk factors, and clinical implications. *Clinical Psychology Review* 18 (7):765–94.

Mackner, L. M., D. P. Sisson, and W. V. Crandall. 2004. Review: Psychosocial issues in pediatric inflammatory bowel disease. *J Pediatr Psychol* 29 (4):243–57.

McDougall, J., G. King, D. J. de Wit, L. T. Miller, S. Hong, D. R. Offord, J. LaPorta, and K. Meyer. 2004. Chronic physical health conditions and disability among Canadian school-aged children: A national profile. *Disabil Rehabil* 26 (1):35–45. doi: 10.1080/09638280410001645076 KKJWLA52C3778ABH [pii].

McQuaid, E. L., S. J. Kopel, and J. H. Nassau. 2001. Behavioral adjustment in children with asthma: a meta-analysis. *J Dev Behav Pediatr* 22 (6):430–39.

Merikangas, K., S. Avenevoli, J. Costello, D. Koretz, and R. C. Kessler. 2009. National comorbidity survey replication adolescent supplement (NCS-A): I. Background and measures. *J Am Acad Child Adolesc Psychiatry* 48 (4):367–69. doi: 10.1097/CHI.0b013e31819996f1.

Merikangas, K. R., H. S. Akiskal, J. Angst, P. E. Greenberg, R. M. Hirschfeld, M. Petukhova, and R. C. Kessler. 2007. Lifetime and 12-month prevalence of bipolar spectrum disorder in the National Comorbidity Survey replication. *Arch Gen Psychiatry* 64 (5):543–52.

Merikangas, K. R., M. Ames, L. Cui, P. E. Stang, T. B. Ustun, M. Von Korff, and R. C. Kessler. 2007. The impact of comorbidity of mental and physical conditions on role disability in the US adult household population. *Arch Gen Psychiatry* 64 (10):1180–88.

Merikangas, K. R., J. P. He, D. Brody, P. W. Fisher, K. Bourdon, and D. S. Koretz. 2010. Prevalence and treatment of mental disorders among US children in the 2001–2004 NHANES. *Pediatrics* 125 (1):75–81. doi: 10.1542/peds.2008-2598peds.2008-2598 [pii].

Merikangas, K. R., J. P. He, M. Burstein, S. A. Swanson, S. Avenevoli, L. Cui, C. Benjet, K. Georgiades, and J. Swendsen. 2010. Lifetime prevalence of mental disorders in U.S. adolescents: results from the National Comorbidity Survey Replication—Adolescent Supplement (NCS-A). *J Am Acad Child Adolesc Psychiatry* 49 (10):980–89. doi: 10.1016/j.jaac.2010.05.017 S0890-8567(10)00476-4 [pii].

Merikangas, K. R., J. P. He, M. Burstein, J. Swendsen, S. Avenevoli, B. Case, K. Georgiades, L. Heaton, S. Swanson, and M. Olfson. 2011. Service utilization for lifetime mental disorders in U.S. adolescents: results of the National Comorbidity Survey-Adolescent Supplement (NCS-A). *J Am Acad Child Adolesc Psychiatry* 50 (1):32–45. doi: 10.1016/j.jaac.2010.10.006 S0890-8567(10)00783-5 [pii].

Merikangas, K. R., J. P. He, J. Rapoport, B. Vitiello, and M. Olfson. 2013. Medication use in US youth with mental disorders. *JAMA Pediatr* 167 (2):141–48. doi: 10.1001/jamapediatrics.2013.431 1465762 [pii].

National Institute of Mental Health. 2001. Report of the National Advisory Mental Health Council's Workgroup on Child and Adolescent Mental Health Intervention Development and Deployment. In *Blueprint for Change: Research on Child and Adolescent Mental Health.*

Ortega, A. N., E. L. McQuaid, G. Canino, R. D. Goodwin, and G. K. Fritz. 2004. Comorbidity of asthma and anxiety and depression in Puerto Rican children. *Psychosomatics* 45 (2):93–99. doi: S0033-3182(04)70202-9 [pii] 10.1176/appi.psy.45.2.93.

Reinherz, H. Z., A. D. Paradis, R. M. Giaconia, C. K. Stashwick, and G. Fitzmaurice. 2003. Childhood and adolescent predictors of major depression in the transition to adulthood. *Am J Psychiatry* 160 (12):2141–47.

Rodenburg, R., G. J. Stams, A. M. Meijer, A. P. Aldenkamp, and M. Dekovic. 2005. Psychopathology in children with epilepsy: A meta-analysis. *J Pediatr Psychol* 30 (6):453–68. doi: jsi071 [pii] 10.1093/jpepsy/jsi071.

Schieve, L. A., S. L. Boulet, C. Boyle, S. A. Rasmussen, and D. Schendel. 2009. Health of children 3 to 17 years of age with Down syndrome in the 1997–2005 national health interview survey. *Pediatrics* 123 (2):e253–60. doi: 10.1542/peds.2008-1440123/2/e253 [pii].

Schwartz, S., and E. Susser. 2006. Commentary: What can epidemiology accomplish? *Int J Epidemiol* 35 (3):587–90; discussion 593–96.

Shaffer, D., P. Fisher, M. K. Dulcan, M. Davies, J. Piacentini, M. E. Schwab-Stone, B. B. Lahey, K. Bourdon, P. S. Jensen, H. R. Bird, G. Canino, and D. A. Regier. 1996. The NIMH Diagnostic Interview Schedule for Children Version 2.3 (DISC-2.3): Description, acceptability, prevalence rates, and performance in the MECA Study. Methods for the Epidemiology of Child and Adolescent Mental Disorders Study. *Journal of the American Academy of Child and Adolescent Psychiatry* 35 (7):865–77.

Shaffer, D., P. Fisher, C. P. Lucas, M. K. Dulcan, and M. E. Schwab-Stone. 2000. NIMH Diagnostic Interview Schedule for Children Version IV (NIMH DISC-IV): Description, differences from previous versions, and reliability of some common diagnoses. *J Am Acad Child Adolesc Psychiatry* 39 (1):28–38.

Simpson, G. A., B. Bloom, R. A. Cohen, S. Blumberg, and K. H. Bourdon. 2005. U.S. children with emotional and behavioral difficulties: data from the 2001, 2002, and 2003 National Health Interview Surveys. *Adv Data* (360):1–13.

Slattery, M. J. 2005. Psychiatric comorbidity associated with atopic disorders in children and adolescents. *Immunol Allergy Clin North Am* 25 (2):407–20, viii. doi: S0889-8561(05)00008-1 [pii] 10.1016/j.iac.2005.02.007.

Spady, D. W., D. P. Schopflocher, L. W. Svenson, and A. H. Thompson. 2005. Medical and psychiatric comorbidity and health care use among children 6 to 17 years old. *Arch Pediatr Adolesc Med* 159 (3):231–37. doi: 159/3/231 [pii] 10.1001/archpedi.159.3.231.

Tsuang, M. T. 2001. Defining alternative phenotypes for genetic studies: What can we learn from studies of schizophrenia? *Am J Med Genet* 105 (1):8–10.

U.S. Department of Health and Human Services. 1999. *Mental Health: A Report of the Surgeon General*. Edited by Substance Abuse and Mental Health Services Administration U.S. Department of Health and Human Services, *Center for Mental Health Services, National Institutes of Health, National Institute of Mental Health*. Rockville, MD.

Weich, S., and R. Araya. 2004. International and regional variation in the prevalence of common mental disorders: Do we need more surveys? *British Journal of Psychiatry* 184:289–290.

Whiteford, H. A., L. Degenhardt, J. Rehm, A. J. Baxter, A. J. Ferrari, H. E. Erskine, F. J. Charlson, R. E. Norman, A. D. Flaxman, N. Johns, R. Burstein, C. J. Murray, and T. Vos. 2013. Global burden of disease attributable to mental and substance use disorders: Findings from the Global Burden of Disease Study 2010. *Lancet*. doi: 10.1016/s0140-6736(13)61611-6.

Wittchen, H. U., C. B. Nelson, and G. Lachner. 1998. Prevalence of mental disorders and psychosocial impairments in adolescents and young adults. *Psychol Med* 28 (1):109–26.

Wu, P., C. W. Hoven, H. R. Bird, R. E. Moore, P. Cohen, M. Alegria, M. K. Dulcan, S. H. Goodman, S. M. Horwitz, J. H. Lichtman, W. E. Narrow, D. S. Rae, D. A. Regier, and M. T. Roper. 1999. Depressive and disruptive disorders and mental health service utilization in children and adolescents. *J Am Acad Child Adolesc Psychiatry* 38 (9):1081–90; discussion 1090–92.

II

PROBLEMS AND DISORDERS

3

Findings and Concepts from Children at Genetic Risk That May Transform Prevention Research and Practice in Schizophrenia and Mood Disorders

Michel Maziade, Elsa Gilbert,
Nicolas Berthelot, and Thomas Paccalet

INTRODUCTION

There is no doubt that new notions and findings about child development are modifying concepts and perceptions of adult major psychiatric disorders particularly affective and non-affective psychotic disorders (Shonkoff et al., 2009; Insel, 2010; Keshavan et al., 2011c; Kahn and Keefe, 2013; Maziade and Paccalet, 2013, 2014). The neurodevelopmental roots of schizophrenia, bipolar disorder, and major depression are emerging as the leading causes of the illnesses and represent the future basis of preventive treatment for these disorders that affect 4 percent of the population. An emerging opinion even reassesses the period of peak incidence for these disorders, i.e., young adulthood, as the treatment-resistant stage of the pathological process and, thus, earlier phases of the disease risk trajectory will constitute the key periods during which different degrees of lighter therapeutic interventions will be effective (McGorry and van Os, 2013). In this chapter we present a selection of findings recently obtained in children and adolescents at risk of psychiatric disorders that supports this encouraging view toward healing these devastating disorders.

We will review the evidence: i) that schizophrenia and mood disorders share several causative mechanisms, and this commonality is already developmentally observable in children at risk; ii) that at-risk children exhibit, early in development, many of the brain functioning anomalies that adult patients display; iii) that the known heterogeneity within adult nosological categories may have its origin in conditions occurring across the childhood-adolescence risk trajectory; and iv) that different combinations of risk factors or risk endophenotypes should be the focus for researchers and clinical practitioners rather than single traits or anomalies.

COMMON CHARACTERISTICS AMONG SCHIZOPHRENIA, BIPOLAR DISORDER, AND MAJOR DEPRESSIVE DISORDER

There are aspects of cognitive or neurophysiological specificity in the endophenotypes, pertaining to schizophrenia or bipolar disorder. However, in terms of public health and prevention these aspects of commonality may have more relevance for and impact upon early detection and preventive treatment of children at risk for both diseases.

It is noteworthy that shared features between schizophrenia and bipolar disorder are increasingly supported by research, including ours (Hill et al., 2008; Lichtenstein et al., 2009; Maziade et al., 2009b; Van Snellenberg and de Candia, 2009; Maziade et al., 2011b), to the point that some have recently recommended combining the two diagnoses to increase the power of genetic studies (Van Snellenberg and de Candia, 2009). We briefly review in the next section the evidence pointing toward shared pathophysiological mechanisms in schizophrenia and bipolar disorder; from clinical manifestations and endophenotypes (cognitive deficits, neurophysiological anomalies) to shared multiple susceptibility genes.

Common Clinical Manifestations

Even though the DSM classification maintains schizophrenia, bipolar disorder, and major depressive disorder in separate entities practicing psychiatrists can attest that differential diagnosis during the first years after disease onset can often prove difficult due to similar clinical symptoms. For instance, during the years following onset, as many as 50 percent of depressive patients will develop manic features that could warrant a change of diagnosis to bipolar disorder (Akiskal, 2009).

Recent articles congruently outline that psychosis and affective symptoms exist on a continuum. For instance, the Bipolar and Schizophrenia Network on Intermediate Phenotypes (B-SNIP) published two studies that clearly suggest a continuous distribution between schizophrenia and psychotic bipolar disorder symptoms (Keshavan et al., 2011b; Tamminga et al., 2013). Keshavan et al. (2011b) assessed the relative proportions of psychotic and affective symptoms over the illness course of 762 patients and concluded that the phenomenological distribution of schizophrenia and bipolar disorder overlapped significantly with 45 percent of patients not corresponding to a prototypical presentation of either disorder.

Another large study from the same group compared the clinical and demographic characteristics of 933 patients with schizophrenia, schizoaffective and bipolar disorder (Tamminga et al., 2013). The findings demonstrate considerable symptom and functioning overlap between the three disorders.

Not only do schizophrenia and bipolar disorder share numerous clinical characteristics but they are also regularly treated with the same medications. For instance, in the B-SNIP study antipsychotics were administered to patients with schizophrenia or bipolar disorder (Tamminga et al., 2013). Moreover, mood stabilizers, which are widely prescribed for bipolar disorder, were reportedly prescribed for more than 20 percent of patients with schizophrenia, while the proportions of patients with schizophrenia or bipolar disorder taking antidepressants were comparable (Tamminga et al., 2013). Thus, it has become common practice for psychiatrists to treat schizophrenia, bipolar disorder and even depression with the same medications leading to the conclusion that the brains of these patients respond, at least in part, to the same treatments.

Shared Cognitive Endophenotypes

A large body of evidence points toward overlapping neuropsychological impairment between schizophrenia, bipolar disorder, and major depressive disorder. Multiple studies have already shown that the three disorders qualitatively share cognitive deficits and present a difference that is mostly quantitative in nature with unipolar and bipolar patient's functioning lying between that of healthy controls and schizophrenia patients (Schretlen et al., 2007; Hill et al., 2008; Maziade et al., 2009b; Reichenberg et al., 2009; Maziade et al., 2011b). For instance, Schretlen et al. (2007) obtained Cohen mean effect sizes of 0.97 across domains for patients with schizophrenia and 0.59 for patients with bipolar disorder. Overall, a continuum of cognitive dysfunction can be observed in schizophrenia and bipolar disorder. Meta-analytic findings document that patients with bipolar disorder outperformed patients with schizophrenia on several cognitive domains such as working memory, verbal memory (immediate and delayed), delayed visual memory, processing speed, executive control, and IQ, whereas in other cognitive domains, such as immediate visual memory and fine motor skills, the impairments of patients with bipolar disorder were in the same range as those with schizophrenia (Krabbendam et al., 2005).

Not surprisingly, recent studies suggest that this continuum in neuropsychological impairment could link schizophrenia to bipolar disorder with psychotic features even more than bipolar disorder without psychosis (Hill et al., 2013). The evidence that neuropsychological deficits may be at the core of schizophrenia and bipolar disorder is supported by the high heritability of such deficits (0.50 to 0.90) (Tuulio-Henriksson et al., 2002; Antila et al., 2007; Horan et al., 2008; Maziade et al., 2011b). Cognitive impairments are not only present in patients but also in non-affected relatives (Tuulio-Henriksson et al., 2003; McIntosh et al., 2005; Snitz et al., 2006; Bora et al., 2009; Maziade et al., 2011b) and in the offspring of patients (Byrne et al., 1999; DelBello and Geller, 2001; Niemi et al., 2003b; Johnstone et al., 2005; Klimes-Dougan et al., 2006; Maziade et al., 2009b; Maziade et al., 2011b) (see "Cognitive Anomalies as Risk Endophenotypes Observed in Childhood" section for more details). Our group recently showed that as many as 25 percent of non-affected adult relatives had at least two cognitive deficits, as defined by a performance under the clinical cut-off below the sixteenth percentile used in neuropsychological practice (Maziade and Paccalet, 2013)

In addition to neurocognitive impairment, the lack of differentiation between schizophrenia and bipolar disorder is supported by an overlap in neurobiological endophenotypes and susceptibility genetic loci (see "Physiological Endophenotype" section). This suggests probable common dysfunctional neurodevelopmental pathways, influenced by genes and environment, leading to major psychiatric disorders (Murray et al., 2004; Maziade et al., 2009b).

Physiological Endophenotypes

Several physiological endophenotypes have been investigated in schizophrenia and mood disorders. Again, even though scientific evidence suggests a degree of inter-diagnosis specificity, schizophrenia, bipolar, and depressive disorders definitely share characteristics.

Electroencephalography/Event-Related Potentials

Electroencephalography (EEG) and related methodologies, such as event-related potentials (ERP), have been intensively studied over the last decades for their propensity to lead to a better understanding of neuropsychiatric disorders. EEG monitoring has the great advantage of being non-invasive and can be performed during normal daily activities through the use of telemetric or ambulatory methods (Leiser et al., 2011). Impairments in EEG and ERP have been widely reported in patients with schizophrenia (Basar and Guntekin, 2008; Leiser et al., 2011) as well as those with bipolar disorder (Lenox et al., 2002; Basar and Guntekin, 2008). Few studies have investigated the overlap of EEG-ERPs anomalies between bipolar disorder and schizophrenia, but scientific evidence already points toward shared anomalies (Thaker, 2008) such as a decreased amplitude of the evoked potential component P300 (Bestelmeyer et al., 2009), auditory ERPs (Rosburg et al., 2008; Jahshan et al., 2012; Ivleva et al., 2013), or ERP related to facial affect processing (Wynn et al., 2013). New concepts have also emerged in schizophrenia (Landgraf and Osterheider, 2013) and bipolar disorder (Maekawa et al., 2013) regarding visual information processing which would be at stake in both illnesses.

Electroretinography

The retina is part of the central nervous system and constitutes a powerful investigation site for understanding brain disorders. The electroretinogram (ERG) is a light-evoked bio-potential recorded on the surface of the eyes (like an EEG) that enables assessment of the full dynamic response originating from the photoreceptors (cones and rods) of the retina. The procedure is non-invasive and without danger for the subject. The ERG waveform is composed of a negative wave called the a-wave generated, for the most part, by the photoreceptors, followed by a more prominent positive component called the b-wave generated by the bipolar cells (see figure 3.1). In an ERG the amplitudes of the a- and b-waves can be easily measured together with other parameters such as the latency of the waveforms (a-wave latency and b-wave latency).

Using the ERG, cone and / or rod anomalies have been reported in disorders such as seasonal affective disorder (Hebert et al., 2002; Hebert et al., 2004; Lavoie et al., 2009), schizophrenia (Warner et al., 1999; Balogh et al., 2008; Hebert et al., Submitted), autism (Ritvo et al., 1988), and Parkinson's disease (Jaffe et al., 1987). Recent findings in youths genetically at risk for schizophrenia and bipolar disorder (Hebert et al., 2010) (see "Physiological Endophenotypes Present in Children" section) have clearly suggested that ERG anomalies would also be present in both schizophrenia and bipolar disorder. These new results can be put in perspective by the findings from ERG studies with adult patients affected by schizophrenia for whom ERG anomalies were found on three of the four parameters of the cone system (a- and b-wave amplitude, and b-wave latency) with effect sizes ranging from 0.47 to 1.32 (Hebert et al., Submitted).

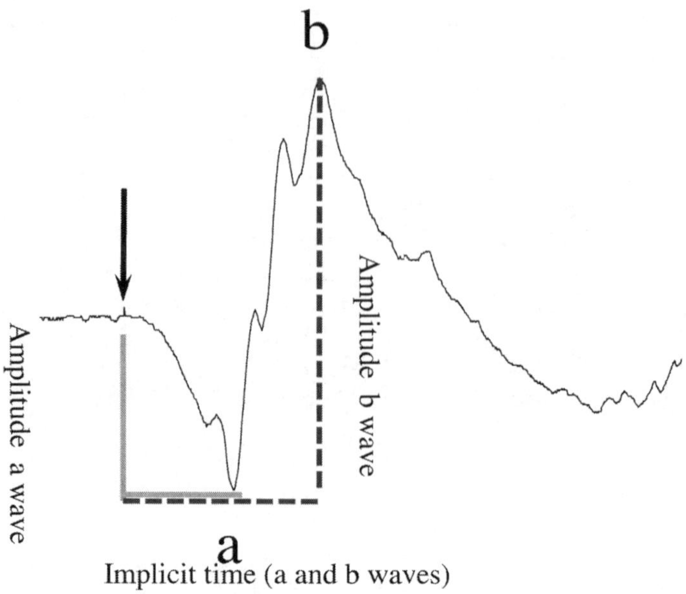

Figure 3.1. Typical electroretinographic response obtained in photopic conditions

Imaging

Brain structures, connectivity and functioning have also been shown to be partly shared in schizophrenia and bipolar disorder. For instance, a recent meta-analysis concluded that regions of the brain showing gray matter reduction were overlapping in bipolar disorder and schizophrenia (Ellison-Wright and Bullmore, 2010). Results of a meta-analysis of magnetic resonance imaging studies (MRI studies) (Arnone et al., 2009) comparing bipolar disorder and schizophrenia indicated that most of the changes in brain volume in bipolar disorder were also observable in schizophrenia. Interestingly, intersecting brain abnormalities among patients with schizophrenia or bipolar disorder have been reported at disease onset suggesting the two disorders share largely overlapping patterns of brain abnormality (De Peri et al., 2012).

Regarding functional MRI studies, overlapping characteristics in schizophrenia and psychotic bipolar disorder can also be found (Khadka et al., 2013).

Candidate Genes and Loci of Risk

There is longstanding evidence for the strong heritability of schizophrenia and bipolar disorder (≈.80) involving multiple liability genes and expression through a host of intermediate and DSM phenotypes (Braff et al., 2007; Szatmari et al., 2007). Several studies suggest that schizophrenia and bipolar disorder share numerous genetic mechanisms as indicated by their familial co-aggregation (Maziade et al., 2005; Lichtenstein et al., 2009; Maziade et al., 2009a; Van Snellenberg and de Candia, 2009) and by several genetic linkage or association signals (Berrettini, 2000b, 2000a; Sklar, 2002; Potash et al., 2003; Maziade et al., 2005; Vazza et al., 2007; Georgieva et al., 2008; Lichtenstein et al., 2009; Purcell et al., 2009). For both disorders genetic linkage analyses have yielded a number of susceptibility loci that converge among studies despite methodological variations and difficulties getting unambiguous confirmation through meta-analysis (Sklar, 2002; Maekawa et al., 2013). As a case in point one recent study (Maekawa et al., 2013) combined independent schizophrenia and bipolar disorder GWAS samples and identified fourteen common loci for these two disorders (out of a total of fifty-eight loci in schizophrenia and thirty-five in bipolar disorders).

It should be noted that genetics common to severe psychiatric disorders are not limited to schizophrenia and bipolar disorder. Two recent studies (Lee et al., 2013; Smoller et al., 2013) provide compelling evidence that major depressive disorder, autism spectrum disorders (ASD) and attention-deficit/hyperactivity disorder (ADHD) share genetic etiology with schizophrenia and bipolar disorder. Such findings support the argument that research in psychiatry would find it advantageous to move beyond individual classical nosological categories and instead investigate common pathophysiologies among different disorders.

In conclusion, the observed high level of continuity between psychotic and mood disorders raises several conceptual and methodological questions for the investigation of the childhood and neurodevelopmental roots of these two disorders.

ENDOPHENOTYPES OF ADULT PATIENTS DETECTABLE EARLY IN CHILDREN AT RISK

The cognitive, physiological, and genetic commonalities between schizophrenia, bipolar disorder, and major depression have led researchers to inquire whether these disorders might share common roots early in the child's development. Recent studies clearly suggest that cognitive and physiological endophenotypes can be found years before prodrome and adult disease incidence, hence suggesting new ways of defining a childhood at-risk cluster or syndrome.

Cognitive Anomalies as Risk Endophenotypes Observed in Childhood

It is now widely acknowledged that cognitive deficits in childhood/adolescence precede the appearance of adult major psychoses. Children at risk of future disease harbor diverse developmental deficits compared to children who remain healthy. For instance, long-term follow-up studies (Erlenmeyer-Kimling et al., 2000; Caspi et al., 2003; Seidman et al., 2006a; Seidman et al., 2006b) found delays in diverse developmental milestones in children who later developed major psychoses. However, conducting longitudinal research in children is difficult, and only a few studies were long-term enough to reach the age of disease incidence of twenty-five to thirty years old (Jones et al. 1994; Cornblatt et al., 1999; Cannon et al., 2000; Erlenmeyer-Kimling et al., 2000; Cannon et al., 2002; Niendam et al., 2003; Osler et al., 2007; Kremen et al., 2010; Reichenberg et al., 2010).

Extensive reviews (Erlenmeyer-Kimling, 2000; Niemi et al., 2003a; Owens and Johnstone, 2006) have confirmed poorer cognitive performance in young at-risk offspring, be it in global IQ (Niendam et al., 2003; Seidman et al., 2006b; Woodberry et al., 2008; Kremen et al., 2010) or specific tasks encompassing attention, memory, and executive functions (Erlenmeyer-Kimling, 2000; Niemi et al., 2003a; Owens and Johnstone, 2006).

Children who develop schizophrenia present a deficit of five to nine points in global IQ (Cannon et al. 2002; Niendam et al. 2003; Seidman et al. 2006b; Woodberry et al. 2008; Kremen et al. 2010). For instance, among the children in the Dunedin birth cohort who developed schizophreniform disorder by age twenty-six, Cannon et al. (2002) reported a fairly stable deficit in global IQ between three to nine years of age along with motor and language delays. Importantly, longitudinal findings about risk trajectories were reported in the same cohort by Reichenberg et al. (2010) and are presented further in the "Developmental Trajectories of Childhood Risk Endophenotypes" section.

When examining specific cognitive domains it appears that at-risk children carry several deficits that are also present in adult patients. For instance, high-risk offspring of parents with schizophrenia have problems in motor and neurological development and poorer performance on executive function, attention, and memory when compared to control children (Byrne et al., 1999; Niemi et al., 2003a). Cognitive deficits are also observed in adolescent offspring of mothers with bipolar disorder compared to offspring of mothers with major depression or controls (Klimes-Dougan et al., 2006), particularly on executive functions and attention which resembles the impairments found in children at high-risk of schizophrenia.

Our group has studied extensively the cognitive functioning of a sample of high-risk offspring of kin suffering from schizophrenia or bipolar disorder in the Eastern Quebec population (Maziade et al., 2009b; Maziade et al., 2011a; Maziade et al., 2011b; Maziade and Paccalet, 2013b). The cognitive deficits observed in these offspring (see Figure 3.2) resemble those reported in children of parents with a sporadic or less familial disease (Byrne et al., 1999; Niemi et al., 2003a; Klimes-Dougan et al., 2006). In terms of inter-disorder commonalities, we also confirmed that impairments in global IQ, episodic memory, and executive functions were similarly present in the offspring of parents with schizophrenia or bipolar disorder (Maziade et al., 2009b). Remarkably, the offspring presented surprisingly large cognitive impairments (as indexed by effect size) when compared to adult patients or along NAARs (Maziade et al., 2009b; Maziade et al., 2011b; Maziade and Paccalet, 2013). In domains like episodic memory, working memory or executive functions the offspring's impairments almost overlapped those of patients (Maziade and Paccalet, 2013).

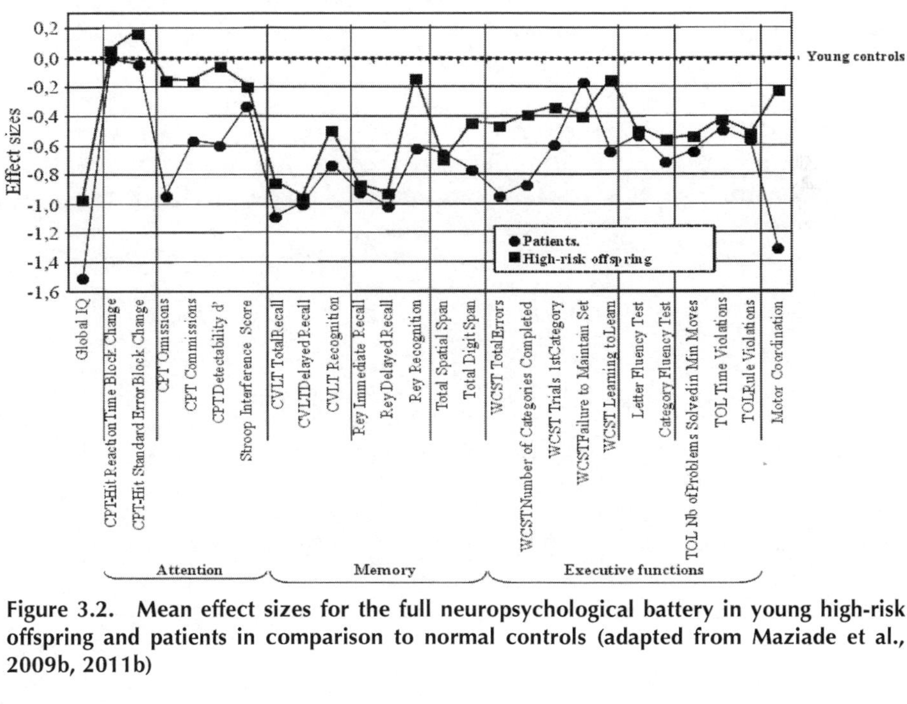

Figure 3.2. Mean effect sizes for the full neuropsychological battery in young high-risk offspring and patients in comparison to normal controls (adapted from Maziade et al., 2009b, 2011b)

Physiological Endophenotypes Present in Children

EEG Anomalies in High-Risk Youth Populations

EEG anomalies in high-risk populations are usually reported in clinically high-risk groups, i.e., youths fitting the ultra high-risk criteria (McGorry et al., 2003). In particular, P300, Mismatch-Negativity (MMN), and P50 anomalies have all been reported in pre-psychotic states (Myles-Worsley et al., 2004; van Tricht et al., 2010; Atkinson et al., 2012; Crossley et al., 2012). As regards the risk for bipolar disorder, fewer studies are available. It is nonetheless suggested that P300 amplitude could also be a valid endophenotype for bipolar disorder since P300 anomalies were detected in unaffected relatives of patients with bipolar disorder (Schulze et al., 2008; Hall et al., 2009).

Few studies have explored EEG/ERP anomalies earlier than the ultra high-risk or prodromal states leaving a dearth of information on the presence of EEG/ERP anomalies years before disease incidence. Recent promising results point toward abnormal pre-attentive auditory event-related potential in subjects across different risk levels of psychotic disorders (Hsieh et al., 2012). For instance, Hsieh et al. (2012) detected mismatch negativity (MMN) deficits even in the group of "early/broad at-risk mental states," i.e., participants at an earlier stage and broader range of at-risk mental states according to Keshavan's definition(Keshavan et al., 2011a).

ERG Anomalies in the Eastern Quebec Kindred Study (EQKS)

ERG has been studied by our group in an Eastern Quebec Kindred Study (EQKS) sample of children/adolescents and young adults at risk for schizophrenia and bipolar disorder. Striking rod response anomalies were found in these young high-risk offspring (Hebert et al., 2010; Maziade and Paccalet, 2013). The differences in rod b-wave amplitude were present both in the offspring of a parent with schizophrenia and those with bipolar disorder. Most importantly, this rod amplitude anomaly was present in both younger (≤ seventeen years) and older offspring (≥ eighteen years; Hebert et al., 2010) diminishing the likelihood of a sole relationship with prodrome and suggesting that ERG anomalies could be childhood precursors of these two disorders. Given the finding in healthy medication-free offspring, our result cannot be attributed to psychopharmacological treatment. Considering that the retina is part of the central nervous system, our data suggest an early dysfunctional process occurring in the brain that, i) is compatible with the schizophrenia neurodevelopmental hypothesis (Hebert et al., 2010), and ii) could represent an early risk biomarker for schizophrenia and bipolar disorder.

DEVELOPMENTAL TRAJECTORIES OF CHILDHOOD RISK ENDOPHENOTYPES

The study of neurodevelopmental endophenotype trajectories in children and adolescents at risk is just beginning, but a few studies already provide insights to orient future research (Cannon et al., 2002; Reichenberg et al., 2010; Maziade et al., 2011a; Maziade and Paccalet, 2013). Tracing such trajectories by using the early cognitive deficits detected in at-risk offspring can provide information with translational implications.

We will focus on two recent studies. First, in the Dunedin cohort, Reichenberg et al. used subtests from the Weschler to follow up 1,037 subjects from age seven to thirteen (Reichenberg et al., 2010) and then reassessed clinical status at age thirty-two. The authors showed two types of cognitive trajectory that distinguished the children who later developed schizophrenia. One trajectory showed a stable developmental delay from age seven to thirteen for verbal acquisitions/reasoning abilities;the second showed a progressive developmental lag from seven to thirteen that was related to processing/visuo-spatial abilities. In other words, two types of cognitive impairment in children at risk exhibited two different trajectories.

In the EQKS study, two datasets led to new concepts for prevention research (Maziade et al., 2011a; Maziade et al., 2011b). Using the framework of multigenerational families affected by schizophrenia or bipolar disorder the observed cognitive functioning in high-risk offspring, adult patients and non-affected adult relatives of patients showed three transgenerational patterns of deficits (see figure 3.3, Maziade et al., 2011b): i) cognitive deficits that were observable only in patients but not in high-risk offspring or non-affected relatives (state markers of disease); ii) deficits that were present in children at risk, patients, and non-affected adult relatives (trait markers that would fit the classical definition of an endophenotype, Braff et al., 2007); and, most relevant, iii) impairments that were present in adult patients and high-risk offspring but not non-affected adult relatives (childhood precursors of disease). These transgenerational patterns of cognitive deficit guided the tracing of cross-sectional trajectories in a large sample of high-risk offspring of severely affected kin (Maziade et al., 2011a).

We observed that the global IQ deficits previously reported in these offspring (Maziade et al., 2009b; Maziade et al., 2011b) was consistently present from primary school years until young adulthood, a result congruent with the meta-analysis of eighteen studies (Woodberry et al., 2008). The EQKS study also analyzed the developmental trajectories of several other cognitive domains including verbal and visual episodic memory and concluded that different cognitive endophenotypes display

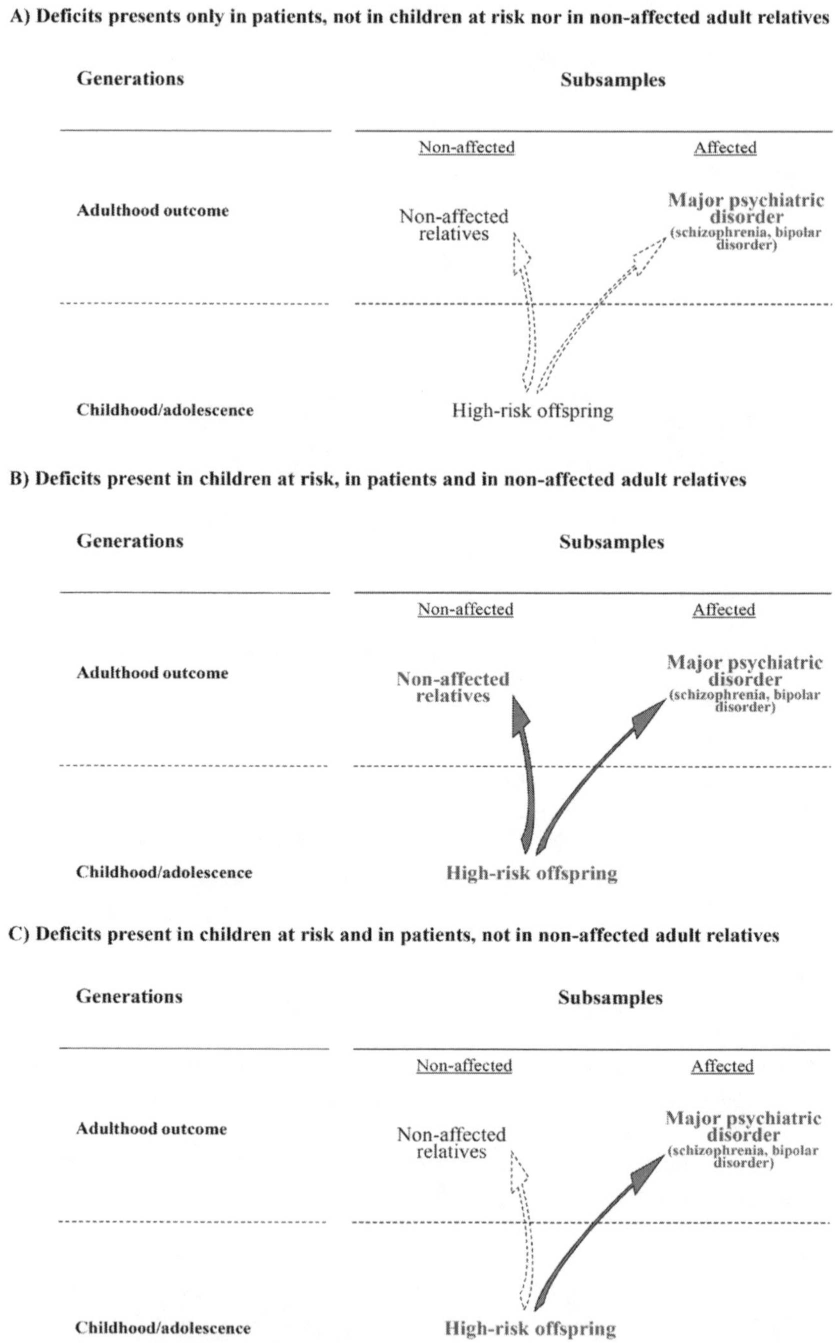

Figure 3.3. Trans-generational patterns of cognitive deficits in young high-risk offspring, adult patients affected by schizophrenia or bipolar disorder, and non-affected adult relatives

different developmental courses (Maziade et al., 2011a; Maziade and Paccalet, 2013), which was somewhat congruent with the Dunedin cohort findings (Reichenberg et al., 2010). Such findings suggest that different risk endophenotypes have different expression timings and this will have implications for targeting the relevant deficits at the right time to define a child as "at risk."

In conclusion, the available data on developmental trajectories in children at risk suggest that differences in developmental patterns may have relevance for prevention research. First, detecting early childhood delays that will remain stable or constant until young adulthood (such as some subtests of IQ or verbal episodic memory) may help the identification of children of higher risk of future disease. However, the presence of a single deficit in a child may not be sufficient to accurately define the future outcome, as discussed below in the next section. Second, more developmentally plastic impairments, i.e., those characterized by deficits that could be unstable along the trajectory, such as some subtests of IQ or visual episodic memory (Reichenberg et al., 2010; Maziade et al., 2011a), suggest that in certain cases the shape of the trajectory across childhood/adolescence may have more meaning than the magnitude of a deficit at any point in the life of the child, as in childhood cardiovascular risk (Barker et al., 2005; Maziade and Paccalet, 2014). Third, the cognitive deficits that only appear after the disease onset or around the prodrome stage might signify impending risk of conversion to a major psychiatric disorder. Novel research methods ought to be applied to the former hypotheses in developmental psychopathology. As an example, a highly relevant question would be whether cognitive remediation should target neuropsychological delays that are more severe rather than those that are more stable across development.

These new findings are encouraging since they are likely to orient future risk and prevention studies toward the crucial goal of targeting the right child, with the right cognitive dysfunction at the right time.

COMBINATIONS OF RISK ENDOPHENOTYPES IN A CHILD MAY HAVE IMPORTANT PREDICTIVE MEANING

Although a single risk factor in childhood is statistically associated with later illness, on its own it might not be sufficient to predict later schizophrenia or bipolar disorder. For instance, we recently showed that a sizeable proportion (up to 25 percent) of the non-affected adult relatives of a patient with schizophrenia or a bipolar patient carried at least two cognitive deficits, based on thresholds accepted in clinical neuropsychology. Comparatively, two or more cognitive deficits were found in only

9.5 percent of the healthy controls whereas 76 percent of the schizophrenia group had such a combination profile (Maziade and Paccalet, 2013). Hence, a single cognitive impairment could not only be a common feature in the general population, but many non-affected adult relatives of patients could present, without ever developing the disease, additional impairments as severely as their affected kin. This observation has led us to devise new hypotheses that are beyond the scope of the present chapter (for more details, see Maziade and Paccalet, 2013).

Cumulative deficits in patients and their relatives are not specific to cognitive impairments and have been observed in many other endophenotypes discovered in schizophrenia and bipolar disorder. The data suggest that the combination of several deficits or risk endophenotypes have a different and better predictive value for the risk of future disease. For instance, the association between impaired cognitive precursors (such as episodic memory) and low social adaptation or attenuated psychosis symptoms in the children of a parent affected by schizophrenia or bipolar disorder is also likely to continue in adult disease (Maziade and Paccalet, 2013) but will be rarer in non-at-risk children.

THE OFFSPRING OF A PARENT AFFECTED BY A MAJOR PSYCHIATRIC DISORDER ARE IN NEED OF CLINICAL HELP IN CHILDHOOD

Rate of Non-Psychotic Behavioral Disorders in Young Offspring at Risk

Given the neurodevelopmental aspects of schizophrenia and bipolar disorders, the investigation of clinical and behavioral deficits in at-risk children have been implemented in an effort to decrypt the clinical precursors of adult psychotic illness. We previously reported that 60 percent of our sample of high-risk offspring descending from multi-affected families presented one or more non-psychotic DSM diagnoses warranting a consultation (i.e., DSM-IV diagnoses that exclude major psychosis or mood disorder) (Maziade et al., 2008). It is noteworthy that this rate is very similar to that reported in several studies of offspring of an affected parent in less familial or sporadic samples (Hans et al., 2004). Diagnoses covered diverse nosological categories (see table 3.1) with a high frequency of comorbid disorders. A British birth cohort also observed that children who later developed schizophrenia presented more internalizing and externalizing behavior disorders, especially anxiety-like behavior (Jones et al., 1994). Intriguingly, we reported that non-psychotic diagnoses had little relation to cognitive dysfunctions (Maziade et al., 2009b).

Table 3.1 Proportions of lifetime DSM-IV diagnoses in the high-risk offspring from densely affected kindreds affected by schizophrenia or bipolar disorder (adapted from Maziade et al. 2008, 2009b)

Lifetime Non-psychotic DSM-IV Diagnoses[a]	*High-risk Offspring Sample*
Any Schizophrenia and Mood Disorders	0
Any Anxiety Disorders	31.1 %
Any Disruptive Disorders	26.7 %
Any Personality Disorders	4.4 %
Learning Disorders	11.1 %
Communication Disorders	4.4 %
Other Disorders	51.1 %
Absence of Diagnosis	37.8 %

[a] Since individuals could have more than one lifetime disorder, the proportions of individual diagnoses do not necessarily add up to 100 percent.

Subclinical or Attenuated Psychotic Symptoms in Children at Risk and in the General Population

Beyond the sole presence of DSM diagnoses in children at risk of adult disease, community sample studies found that psychotic-like experiences were frequent in the general population. For instance, 5–8 percent of adults in the general population had experienced at least one psychotic symptom in an attenuated form (Kelleher et al., 2010). Similarly, prospective population-based cohorts also indicated that 5–6 percent of children displayed psychotic symptoms in a sub-threshold or attenuated form early in life (Laurens et al., 2007; Polanczyk et al., 2010). Genetically at risk children from the EQKS sample had a comparable rate of psychotic-like symptoms in an attenuated form (unpublished data).

Subclinical psychotic experiences in the general population are usually transitory. It is the persistence of such attenuated symptoms that could increase the likelihood of later psychotic disorder (van Os et al., 2009; Dominguez et al., 2011). However, there is a complex longitudinal relationship between childhood attenuated psychotic symptoms and later occurrence of a psychotic disorder. Indeed, only 20 percent of children reporting attenuated symptoms in childhood later developed a psychotic disorder, whereas 50 percent of adult patients reported attenuated symptoms during childhood (Poulton et al., 2000; Ruhrmann et al., 2010). These findings highlight that early sub-threshold clinical symptoms may be the expression of an underlying liability but the causative mechanisms require further study.

Childhood Trauma as an Aggravating Risk Factor

Childhood trauma has indisputably come to the foreground of schizophrenia research in recent years. Recent research supports the causal relationship between trauma and psychosis (Kelleher et al., 2013). Patients with psychosis are almost three times more likely to be exposed in early life to abuse or neglect than healthy controls, and trauma exposure could potentially explain a third of psychotic illness incidence (Varese et al., 2012b). The association with trauma holds both for schizophrenia (Read et al., 2005; Varese et al., 2012b) and bipolar disorder (Leverich and Post, 2006; Larsson et al., 2013), again suggesting common vulnerability due to serious stressful experiences in childhood.

The impact of trauma on child and adolescent development could take different forms. *First,* trauma exposure might interfere with brain maturational processes. Early life adversity is suggested to hyperactivate the neural circuits of the hypothalamic-pituitary-adrenal (HPA) axis and to impinge on the brain structures (Heim et al., 2010; Juster et al., 2011) that are documented as affected in patients with psychosis, such as the hippocampus (Adriano et al., 2012). *Second,* some of the childhood cognitive deficits could be partly attributed to trauma exposure. For instance, children at high genetic risk exposed to abuse or neglect were much more likely to present visual episodic memory deficits than high-risk offspring without trauma history (Berthelot et al. Submitted). Childhood trauma was similarly associated with cognitive impairments in adults with psychosis (Schenkel et al., 2005; Aas et al., 2011; Shannon et al., 2011). *Third,* childhood trauma interferes with early attachment relationships. Such disturbed caregiver-child relationships may result in disorganized working models of attachment (Cyr et al., 2010; Alexander, 2013) and interfere with the acquisition of mentalization (Fonagy et al., 2011). Unresolved/disorganized attachment and poor mentalization/metacognitive abilities are suggested to play a role in the development of psychosis (Liotti and Gumley, 2008). *Fourth,* children exposed to trauma commonly develop clinical symptoms in the short term such as dissociation (Hulette et al., 2011; Bernier et al., 2013). Dissociation may mediate the relationship between trauma exposure and externalizing and internalizing problems (Collin-Vezina and Hebert, 2005; Berthelot et al., 2012) as well as psychotic symptoms (Steingard and Frankel, 1985; Varese et al., 2012a; Braehler et al., 2013).

These different mechanisms should be seen as the result of complex interactions between trauma characteristics (such as the subjective experience, the degree of severity and timing of the trauma) and the individual's past development and genetic predispositions. From a neurobiological, neurocognitive, attachment, or clinical perspective, one conclusion stands out: the risk-effect of trauma in schizophrenia and mood disorder cannot be ignored in risk and prevention studies, and it has immediate implications for public health priorities and mental health daily practice regarding the vulnerability to major psychiatric disorders.

FROM RESEARCH TO PRACTICE

Chapter Summary

In this chapter, we reviewed key findings suggesting critical developmental pathophysiological mechanisms that are likely to predispose a child to schizophrenia or mood disorders. First, we reviewed the clinical, cognitive, neurophysiological, and imaging commonalities between both diseases. We also noted that even from a genetic standpoint numerous susceptibility loci were shared by schizophrenia and bipolar disorder. We then focused on the children at risk of future disease and observed that most of the cognitive and neurophysiological anomalies (that we called risk endophenotypes) and carried by adult patients can also be detected in children many years before disease incidence. We proposed that risk endophenotypes have a longitudinal course and that examining the shape of these developmental trajectories may be relevant for risk assessment and prevention above and beyond the presence of a risk endophenotype at any single moment along the trajectory. In parallel, the accummulation of deficits may also have a special predictive significance in terms of disease risk. Indeed, children at risk and non-affected adult relatives of patients exihibit combinations of deficits more frequently than individuals in the general population. Independent of risk, we raised the issue that the children at risk of schizophrenia and bipolar disorder develop behavioral and developmental problems that call for immediate clinical attention from the practitioner. Finally, childhood exposure to abuse and neglect is definitely related to later adult incidence of psychotic and mood disorders and this fact has compelling consequences for the practice of child psychologists, psychiatrists, and allied professions.

The new concepts reviewed in this chapter are emerging at a time when schizophrenia research calls for new models and thinking "outside the box" (Insel, 2010; Keshavan et al., 2011c; Maziade and Paccalet, 2013); the developmental discoveries in schizophrenia and bipolar disorder will change our view of the causes of and treatment for these devastating illnesses.

Conclusion: Novel Ways and Methods to Reinvent Developmental Research in Major Psychiatric Disorders

Developmental research in at-risk children and adolescents is likely to become the new route to discovery. Known obstacles to research in adult disorders may have their roots in the childhood risk trajectory. A good example is the disease's widespread heterogeneity. Keshavan et al. (2011c) have advocated that heterogeneity should not be an excuse for the scientific community's lack of breakthroughs; to the contrary, it should be the problem to be solved. A good way to address heterogeneity may be to look for events or anomalies in the longitudinal trajectory of vulnerable children that could explain phenotypic and outcome variability among adult patients. Second, rather than being an obstacle, the established commonalities between schizophrenia and mood disorders might also be assets from a developmental viewpoint. Scientists may conceive that there is a common childhood "syndrome at-risk," made up of different combinations of risk endophenotypes that would be pluripotent in terms of adult outcome dependent on the gene-environment events occurring at different times along the trajectory (McGorry and van Os, 2013). Hence, increasing evidence suggests that risk factors and mechanisms, as well as the characteristics of childhood risk trajectories, may be common to different sets of complex brain and physical disorders (Brent and Silverstein, 2013; Maziade and Paccalet, 2014). In addition to a rapprochement with cancer research (Maziade and Paccalet, 2013b) we recently proposed that metabolic-cardiovascular disorders shared causative attributes not only in adulthood but also in childhood (Maziade and Paccalet, 2014). For instance, childhood trauma could predict both psychiatric disorders and cardiac incidents in adulthood due to still unknown shared mechanisms. The search for such shared mechanisms may accelerate our understanding of the causative processes and transform our notion of etiology, prevention and curative treatment. Admittedly, investigating the roots of major psychiatric disorders and other complex diseases in tandem is part of an emerging international scientific consensus (Shonkoff et al., 2009) that the origins of most adult diseases are found in developmental and biological aberrancies occurring during the early years of life.

REFERENCES

Aas, M., Dazzan, P., et al. 2011. Childhood trauma and cognitive function in first-episode affective and non-affective psychosis. *Schizophrenia Research* 129 (1):12–19.

Adriano, F., Caltagirone, C., et al. 2012. Hippocampal volume reduction in first-episode and chronic schizophrenia: a review and meta-analysis. *Neuroscientist* 18 (2):180–200.

Akiskal, H. S. 2009. Mood Disorders. In *Kaplan and Sadock's Comprehensive Textbook of Psychiatry*, edited by B. J. Sadock, V. A. Sadock, and P. Ruiz: Lippincott Williams & Wilkins (LWW).

Alexander, P. C. 2013. Relational trauma and disorganized attachment. Edited by J. D. Ford and C. A. Courtois, *Treating Complex Traumatic Stress Disorders in Children and Adolescents*. New York: Guildford Press.

Antila, M., Tuulio-Henriksson, A., et al. 2007. Heritability of cognitive functions in families with bipolar disorder. *Am J Med Genet B Neuropsychiatr Genet* 144B (6):802–8.

Arnone, D., Cavanagh, J., et al. 2009. Magnetic resonance imaging studies in bipolar disorder and schizophrenia: meta-analysis. *Br J Psychiatry* 195 (3):194–201.

Atkinson, R. J., Michie, P. T., et al. 2012. Duration mismatch negativity and P3a in first-episode psychosis and individuals at ultra-high risk of psychosis. *Biol Psychiatry* 71 (2):98–104.

Balogh, Z., Benedek, G., et al. 2008. Retinal dysfunctions in schizophrenia. *Prog Neuropsychopharmacol Biol Psychiatry* 32 (1):297–300.

Barker, D. J., Osmond, C., et al. 2005. Trajectories of growth among children who have coronary events as adults. *N Engl J Med* 353 (17):1802–9.

Basar, E., and Guntekin, B. 2008. A review of brain oscillations in cognitive disorders and the role of neurotransmitters. *Brain Research* 1235:172–93.

Bernier, M. J., Hebert, M., et al. 2013. Dissociative symptoms over a year in a sample of sexually abused children. *J Trauma Dissociation* 14 (4):455–72.

Berrettini, W. H. 2000a. Are schizophrenic and bipolar disorders related? A review of family and molecular studies. *Biol Psychiatry* 48 (6):531–38.

Berrettini, W. H. 2000b. Susceptibility loci for bipolar disorder: Overlap with inherited vulnerability to schizophrenia. *Biol Psychiatry* 47 (3):245–51.

Berthelot, N., Maheux, J., et al. 2012. The mediating role of dissociation in the association between childhood sexual abuse and clinical symptomatology / La dissociation comme médiateur entre l'agression sexuelle et la symptomatologie clinique chez l'enfant. *Revue Québécoise de Psychologie* 33 (3):37–58.

Berthelot, N., Paccalet, T., et al. Submitted. Mediating mechanisms and temporality in the adverse effect of childhood trauma on childhood cognitive precursors of major psychiatric disorders.

Bestelmeyer, P. E., Phillips, L. H., et al. 2009. The P300 as a possible endophenotype for schizophrenia and bipolar disorder: Evidence from twin and patient studies. *Psychiatry Res* 169 (3):212–19.

Bora, E., Yucel, M., et al. 2009. Cognitive endophenotypes of bipolar disorder: A meta-analysis of neuropsychological deficits in euthymic patients and their first-degree relatives. *J Affect Disord* 113 (1-2):1–20.

Braehler, C., Valiquette, L., et al. 2013. Childhood trauma and dissociation in first-episode psychosis, chronic schizophrenia and community controls. *Psychiatry Res*.

Braff, D. L., Freedman, R., et al. 2007. Deconstructing schizophrenia: an overview of the use of endophenotypes in order to understand a complex disorder. *Schizophr Bull* 33 (1):21–32.

Brent, D. A., and Silverstein, M. 2013. Shedding light on the long shadow of childhood adversity. *JAMA* 309 (17):1777–78.

Byrne, M., Hodges, A., et al. 1999. Neuropsychological assessment of young people at high genetic risk for developing schizophrenia compared with controls:

Preliminary findings of the Edinburgh High Risk Study (EHRS). *Psychological Medicine* 29 (5):1161–73.

Cannon, M., Caspi, A., et al. 2002. Evidence for early-childhood, pan-developmental impairment specific to schizophreniform disorder: results from a longitudinal birth cohort. *Arch Gen Psychiatry* 59 (5):449–56.

Cannon, T. D., Bearden, C. E., et al. 2000. Childhood cognitive functioning in schizophrenia patients and their unaffected siblings: A prospective cohort study. *Schizophr Bull* 26 (2):379–93.

Caspi, A., Reichenberg, A., et al. 2003. Cognitive performance in schizophrenia patients assessed before and following the first psychotic episode. *Schizophr Res* 65 (2–3):87–94.

Collin-Vezina, D., and Hebert, M. 2005. Comparing dissociation and PTSD in sexually abused school-aged girls. *J Nerv Ment Dis* 193 (1):47–52.

Cornblatt, B., Obuchowski, M., et al. 1999. Cognitive and behavioral precursors of schizophrenia. *Developmental Psychopathology* 11 (3):487–508.

Crossley, N.A., Constante, M., et al. 2012. Neurophysiological alterations in the prepsychotic phases. *Curr Pharm Des* 18 (4):479–85.

Cyr, C., Euser, E. M., et al. 2010. Attachment security and disorganization in maltreating and high-risk families: a series of meta-analyses. *Dev Psychopathol* 22 (1):87–108.

De Peri, L., Crescini, A., et al. 2012. Brain structural abnormalities at the onset of schizophrenia and bipolar disorder: A meta-analysis of controlled magnetic resonance imaging studies. *Curr Pharm Des* 18 (4):486–94.

DelBello, M. P., and Geller, B. 2001. Review of studies of child and adolescent offspring of bipolar parents. *Bipolar Disorders* 3 (6):325–334.

Dominguez, M. D., Wichers, M., et al. 2011. Evidence that onset of clinical psychosis is an outcome of progressively more persistent subclinical psychotic experiences: An 8-year cohort study. *Schizophr Bull* 37 (1):84–93.

Ellison-Wright, I., and Bullmore, E. 2010. Anatomy of bipolar disorder and schizophrenia: A meta-analysis. *Schizophr Res* 117 (1):1–12.

Erlenmeyer-Kimling, L. 2000. Neurobehavioral deficits in offspring of schizophrenic parents: Liability indicators and predictors of illness. *American Journal of Medical Genetics* 97 (1):65–71.

Erlenmeyer-Kimling, L., Rock, D., et al. 2000. Attention, memory, and motor skills as childhood predictors of schizophrenia-related psychoses: the New York High-Risk Project. *Am J Psychiatry* 157 (9):1416–22.

Fonagy, P., Luyten, P., et al. 2011. Borderline Personality Disorder, Mentalization, and the Neurobiology of Attachment. *Infant Mental Health Journal* 32 (1):47–69.

Georgieva, L., Dimitrova, A., et al. 2008. Support for neuregulin 1 as a susceptibility gene for bipolar disorder and schizophrenia. *Biol Psychiatry* 64 (5):419–27.

Hall, M.H., Schulze, K., et al. 2009. Are auditory P300 and duration MMN heritable and putative endophenotypes of psychotic bipolar disorder? A Maudsley Bipolar Twin and Family Study. *Psychol Med* 39 (8):1277–87.

Hans, S. L., Auerbach, J. G., et al. 2004. Offspring of parents with schizophrenia: Mental disorders during childhood and adolescence. *Schizophrenia Bulletin* 30 (2):303–15.

Hebert, M., Beattie, C., et al. 2004. Electroretinography in patients with winter seasonal affective disorder. *Psychiatry Research* 127:27–34.
Hebert, M., Dumont, M., et al. 2002. Electrophysiological evidence suggesting a seasonal modulation of retinal sensitivity in subsyndromal winter depression. *J Affect Disord* 68 (2-3):191–202.
Hebert, M., Gagne, A. M., et al. 2010. Retinal response to light in young nonaffected offspring at high genetic risk of neuropsychiatric brain disorders. *Biol Psychiatry* 67 (3):270–74.
Hebert, M., Merette, C., et al. Submitted. Electroretinographic profile distinghuishes schizophrenia from healthy subjects: Prospects for disease biomarkers.
Heim, C., Shugart, M., et al. 2010. Neurobiological and psychiatric consequences of child abuse and neglect. *Dev Psychobiol* 52 (7):671–90.
Hill, S. K., Harris, M. S., et al. 2008. Neurocognitive allied phenotypes for schizophrenia and bipolar disorder. *Schizophr Bull* 34 (4):743–59.
Hill, S. K., Reilly, J. L., et al. 2013. Neuropsychological Impairments in Schizophrenia and Psychotic Bipolar Disorder: Findings from the Bipolar and Schizophrenia Network on Intermediate Phenotypes (B-SNIP) Study. *Am J Psychiatry.*
Horan, W. P., Braff, D. L., et al. 2008. Verbal working memory impairments in individuals with schizophrenia and their first-degree relatives: Findings from the Consortium on the Genetics of Schizophrenia. *Schizophr Res* 103 (1–3):218–28.
Hsieh, M. H., Shan, J. C., et al. 2012. Auditory event-related potential of subjects with suspected pre-psychotic state and first-episode psychosis. *Schizophr Res* 140 (1–3):243–49.
Hulette, A. C., Freyd, J. J., et al. 2011. Dissociation in middle childhood among foster children with early maltreatment experiences. *Child Abuse Negl* 35 (2):123–26.
Insel, T. R. 2010. Rethinking schizophrenia. *Nature* 468 (7321):187–93.
Ivleva, E. I., Moates, A. F., et al. 2013. Smooth pursuit eye movement, prepulse inhibition, and auditory paired stimuli processing endophenotypes across the schizophrenia-bipolar disorder psychosis dimension. *Schizophrenia Bulletin.*
Jaffe, M. J., Bruno, G., et al. 1987. Ganzfeld electroretinographic findings in parkinsonism: untreated patients and the effect of levodopa intravenous infusion. *J Neurol Neurosurg Psychiatry* 50 (7):847–52.
Jahshan, C., Wynn, J. K., et al. 2012. Cross-diagnostic comparison of duration mismatch negativity and P3a in bipolar disorder and schizophrenia. *Bipolar Disord* 14 (3):239–48.
Johnstone, E. C., Ebmeier, K. P., et al. 2005. Predicting schizophrenia: Findings from the Edinburgh high-risk study. *British Journal of Psychiatry* 186:18–25.
Jones, P., Rodgers, B., et al. 1994. Child development risk factors for adult schizophrenia in the British 1946 birth cohort. *Lancet* 344 (8934):1398–402.
Juster, R. P., Bizik, G., et al. 2011. A transdisciplinary perspective of chronic stress in relation to psychopathology throughout life span development. *Dev Psychopathol* 23 (3):725–76.
Kahn, R. S., and Keefe, R. S. 2013. Schizophrenia is a cognitive illness: Time for a change in focus. *JAMA Psychiatry.*
Kelleher, I., Jenner, J. A., et al. 2010. Psychotic symptoms in the general population—an evolutionary perspective. *British Journal of Psychiatry* 197 (3):167–69.

Kelleher, I., Keeley, H., et al. 2013. Childhood trauma and psychosis in a prospective cohort study: Cause, effect, and directionality. *American Journal of Psychiatry* 170 (7):734–41.

Keshavan, M. S., DeLisi, L. E., et al. 2011a. Early and broadly defined psychosis risk mental states. *Schizophr Res* 126 (1–3):1–10.

Keshavan, M. S., Morris, D. W., et al. 2011b. A dimensional approach to the psychosis spectrum between bipolar disorder and schizophrenia: The schizo-bipolar scale. *Schizophr Res* 133 (1–3):250–54.

Keshavan, M. S., Nasrallah, H. A., et al. 2011c. Schizophrenia, just the facts 6. Moving ahead with the schizophrenia concept: From the elephant to the mouse. *Schizophr Res* 127 (1–3):3-13.

Khadka, S., Meda, S. A., et al. 2013. Is aberrant functional connectivity a psychosis endophenotype? A resting state functional magnetic resonance imaging study. *Biological Psychiatry* 74 (6):458–66.

Klimes-Dougan, B., Ronsaville, D., et al. 2006. Neuropsychological functioning in adolescent children of mothers with a history of bipolar or major depressive disorders. *Biol Psychiatry* 60 (9):957–65.

Krabbendam, L., Arts, B., et al. 2005. Cognitive functioning in patients with schizophrenia and bipolar disorder: A quantitative review. *Schizophr Res* 80 (2–3):137–49.

Kremen, W. S., Vinogradov, S., et al. 2010. Cognitive decline in schizophrenia from childhood to midlife: A 33-year longitudinal birth cohort study. *Schizophr Res* doi:10.1016/j.schres.2010.01.009.

Landgraf, S., and Osterheider, M. 2013. To see or not to see: That is the question. The Protection-Against-Schizophrenia (PaSZ) model: Evidence from congenital blindness and visuo-cognitive aberrations. *Front Psychol* 4:352.

Larsson, S., Andreassen, O. A., et al. 2013. High prevalence of childhood trauma in patients with schizophrenia spectrum and affective disorder. *Compr Psychiatry* 54 (2):123–27.

Laurens, K. R., Hodgins, S., et al. 2007. Community screening for psychotic-like experiences and other putative antecedents of schizophrenia in children aged 9–12 years. *Schizophr Res* 90 (1–3):130–46.

Lavoie, M. P., Lam, R. W., et al. 2009. Evidence of a biological effect of light therapy on the retina of patients with seasonal affective disorder. *Biological Psychiatry* 66 (3):253–58.

Lee, S. H., Ripke, S., et al. 2013. Genetic relationship between five psychiatric disorders estimated from genome-wide SNPs. *Nature Genetics*.

Leiser, S. C., Dunlop, J., et al. 2011. Aligning strategies for using EEG as a surrogate biomarker: A review of preclinical and clinical research. *Biochem Pharmacol* 81 (12):1408–21.

Lenox, R. H., Gould, T. D., et al. 2002. Endophenotypes in bipolar disorder. *American Journal of Medical Genetics* 114 (4):391–406.

Leverich, G. S., and Post, R. M. 2006. Course of bipolar illness after history of childhood trauma. *Lancet* 367 (9516):1040–42.

Lichtenstein, P., Yip, B. H., et al. 2009. Common genetic determinants of schizophrenia and bipolar disorder in Swedish families: A population-based study. *Lancet* 373 (9659):234–39.

Liotti, G., and Gumley, A. 2008. An attachment perspective on schizophrenia: Disorganized attachment, dissociative processes, and compromised mentalisation. In *Dissociation and psychosis: Converging perspectives on a complex relationship*, edited by A. Moskowitz, M. Dorahy, and I. Schaefer. Hoboken, NJ: Wiley.

Maekawa, T., Katsuki, S., et al. 2013. Altered visual information processing systems in bipolar disorder: Evidence from visual MMN and P3. *Front Hum Neurosci* 7:403.

Maziade, M., Chagnon, Y. C., et al. 2009a. Chromosome 13q13-q14 locus overlaps mood and psychotic disorders: The relevance for redefining phenotype. *Eur J Hum Genet* 17 (8):1034–42.

Maziade, M., Gingras, N., et al. 2008. Clinical diagnoses in young offspring from eastern Quebec multigenerational families densely affected by schizophrenia or bipolar disorder. *Acta Psychiatr Scand* 117 (2):118–26.

Maziade, M., and Paccalet, T. 2014. Common determinants of psychiatric and cardiovascular disorders call for common prevention and clinical research. *JAMA Pediatrics* 168 (1):3–4.

Maziade, M., and Paccalet, T. 2013. A protective-compensatory model may reconcile the genetic and the developmental findings in schizophrenia. *Schizophr Res* 144 (1–3):9–15.

Maziade, M., Rouleau, N., et al. 2011a. Young offspring at genetic risk of adult psychoses: The form of the trajectory of IQ or memory may orient to the right dysfunction at the right time. *PLoS One* 6 (4):e19153.

Maziade, M., Rouleau, N., et al. 2011b. Verbal and visual memory impairments among young offspring and healthy adult relatives of patients with schizophrenia and bipolar disorder: Selective generational patterns indicate different developmental trajectories. *Schizophr Bull* 37 (6):1218–28.

Maziade, M., Rouleau, N., et al. 2009b. Shared neurocognitive dysfunctions in young offspring at extreme risk for schizophrenia or bipolar disorder in eastern quebec multigenerational families. *Schizophrenia Bulletin* 35 (5):919–30.

Maziade, M., Roy, M. A., et al. 2005. Shared and specific susceptibility loci for schizophrenia and bipolar disorder: A dense genome scan in Eastern Quebec families. *Mol Psychiatry* 10 (5):486–99.

McGorry, P., and van Os, J. 2013. Redeeming diagnosis in psychiatry: Timing versus specificity. *Lancet* 381 (9863):343–45.

McGorry, P. D., Yung, A. R., et al. 2003. The 'close-in' or ultra high-risk model: A safe and effective strategy for research and clinical intervention in prepsychotic mental disorder. *Schizophr Bull* 29 (4):771–90.

McIntosh, A. M., Harrison, L. K., et al. 2005. Neuropsychological impairments in people with schizophrenia or bipolar disorder and their unaffected relatives. *Br J Psychiatry* 186:378–85.

Murray, R. M., Sham, P., et al. 2004. A developmental model for similarities and dissimilarities between schizophrenia and bipolar disorder. *Schizophr Res* 71 (2–3):405–16.

Myles-Worsley, M., Ord, L., et al. 2004. P50 sensory gating in adolescents from a pacific island isolate with elevated risk for schizophrenia. *Biol Psychiatry* 55 (7):663–67.

Niemi, L. T., Suvisaari, J. M., et al. 2003a. Childhood developmental abnormalities in schizophrenia: Evidence from high-risk studies. *Schizophr Res* 60 (2–3):239–58.
Niemi, L. T., Suvisaari, J. M., et al. 2003b. Childhood developmental abnormalities in schizophrenia: Evidence from high-risk studies. *Schizophrenia Research* 60:239–58.
Niendam, T. A., Bearden, C. E., et al. 2003. A prospective study of childhood neurocognitive functioning in schizophrenic patients and their siblings. *American Journal of Psychiatry* 160 (11):2060–62.
Osler, M., Lawlor, D. A., et al. 2007. Cognitive function in childhood and early adulthood and hospital admission for schizophrenia and bipolar disorders in Danish men born in 1953. *Schizophr Res* 92 (1–3):132–41.
Owens, D. G., and Johnstone, E. C. 2006. Precursors and prodromata of schizophrenia: Findings from the Edinburgh High Risk Study and their literature context. *Psychological Medicine* 36 (11):1501–14.
Polanczyk, G., Moffitt, T. E., et al. 2010. Etiological and clinical features of childhood psychotic symptoms: Results from a birth cohort. *Arch Gen Psychiatry* 67 (4):328–38.
Potash, J. B., Zandi, P. P., et al. 2003. Suggestive linkage to chromosomal regions 13q31 and 22q12 in families with psychotic bipolar disorder. *American Journal of Psychiatry* 160 (4):680–686.
Poulton, R., Caspi, A., et al. 2000. Children's self-reported psychotic symptoms and adult schizophreniform disorder: A 15-year longitudinal study. *Arch Gen Psychiatry* 57 (11):1053–58.
Purcell, S. M., Wray, N. R., et al. 2009. Common polygenic variation contributes to risk of schizophrenia and bipolar disorder. *Nature* 460 (7256):748–52.
Read, J., van Os, J., et al. 2005. Childhood trauma, psychosis and schizophrenia: A literature review with theoretical and clinical implications. *Acta Psychiatr Scand* 112 (5):330–50.
Reichenberg, A., Caspi, A., et al. 2010. Static and dynamic cognitive deficits in childhood preceding adult schizophrenia: A 30-year study. *American Journal of Psychiatry* 167 (2):160–69.
Reichenberg, A., Harvey, P. D., et al. 2009. Neuropsychological function and dysfunction in schizophrenia and psychotic affective disorders. *Schizophrenia Bulletin* 35 (5):1022–29.
Ritvo, E. R., Creel, D., et al. 1988. Electroretinograms in autism: a pilot study of b-wave amplitudes. *Am J Psychiatry* 145 (2):229–32.
Rosburg, T., Boutros, N. N., et al. 2008. Reduced auditory evoked potential component N100 in schizophrenia—a critical review. *Psychiatry Res* 161 (3):259–74.
Ruhrmann, S., Schultze-Lutter, F., et al. 2010. Prediction of psychosis in adolescents and young adults at high risk: Results from the prospective European prediction of psychosis study. *Arch Gen Psychiatry* 67 (3):241–51.
Schenkel, L. S., Spaulding, W. D., et al. 2005. Histories of childhood maltreatment in schizophrenia: Relationships with premorbid functioning, symptomatology, and cognitive deficits. *Schizophr Res* 76 (2–3):273–86.
Schretlen, D. J., Cascella, N. G., et al. 2007. Neuropsychological functioning in bipolar disorder and schizophrenia. *Biol Psychiatry* 62 (2):179–86.

Schulze, K. K., Hall, M. H., et al. 2008. Auditory P300 in patients with bipolar disorder and their unaffected relatives. *Bipolar Disord* 10 (3):377–86.

Seidman, L. J., Buka, S. L., et al. 2006a. Intellectual decline in schizophrenia: Evidence from a prospective birth cohort 28 year follow-up study. *J Clin Exp Neuropsychol* 28 (2):225–42.

Seidman, L. J., Giuliano, A. J., et al. 2006b. Neuropsychological functioning in adolescents and young adults at genetic risk for schizophrenia and affective psychoses: Results from the Harvard and Hillside Adolescent High Risk Studies. *Schizophr Bull* 32 (3):507–24.

Shannon, C., Douse, K., et al. 2011. The association between childhood trauma and memory functioning in schizophrenia. *Schizophr Bull* 37 (3):531–37.

Shonkoff, J. P., Boyce, W. T., et al. 2009. Neuroscience, molecular biology, and the childhood roots of health disparities: Building a new framework for health promotion and disease prevention. *Jama* 301 (21):2252–59.

Sklar, P. 2002. Linkage analysis in psychiatric disorders: The emerging picture. *Annu Rev Genomics Hum Genet* 3:371–413.

Smoller, J. W., Craddock, N., et al. 2013. Identification of risk loci with shared effects on five major psychiatric disorders: A genome-wide analysis. *Lancet* 381 (9875):1371–79.

Snitz, B. E., Macdonald, A. W., 3rd, et al. 2006. Cognitive deficits in unaffected first-degree relatives of schizophrenia patients: A meta-analytic review of putative endophenotypes. *Schizophr Bull* 32 (1):179–94.

Steingard, S., and Frankel, F. H. 1985. Dissociation and psychotic symptoms. *Am J Psychiatry* 142 (8):953–55.

Szatmari, P., Maziade, M., et al. 2007. Informative phenotypes for genetic studies of psychiatric disorders. *Am J Med Genet B Neuropsychiatr Genet* 144 (5):581–88.

Tamminga, C. A., Ivleva, E. I., et al. 2013. Clinical Phenotypes of Psychosis in the Bipolar and Schizophrenia Network on Intermediate Phenotypes (B-SNIP). *Am J Psychiatry*.

Thaker, G. K. 2008. Neurophysiological endophenotypes across bipolar and schizophrenia psychosis. *Schizophrenia Bulletin* 34 (4):760–73.

Tuulio-Henriksson, A., Arajarvi, R., et al. 2003. Familial loading associates with impairment in visual span among healthy siblings of schizophrenia patients. *Biol Psychiatry* 54 (6):623–28.

Tuulio-Henriksson, A., Haukka, J., et al. 2002. Heritability and number of quantitative trait loci of neurocognitive functions in families with schizophrenia. *Am J Med Genet* 114 (5):483–90.

van Os, J., Linscott, R. J., et al. 2009. A systematic review and meta-analysis of the psychosis continuum: Evidence for a psychosis proneness-persistence-impairment model of psychotic disorder. *Psychol Med* 39 (2):179–95.

Van Snellenberg, J. X., and de Candia, T. 2009. Meta-analytic evidence for familial coaggregation of schizophrenia and bipolar disorder. *Arch Gen Psychiatry* 66 (7):748–55.

van Tricht, M. J., Nieman, D. H., et al. 2010. Reduced parietal P300 amplitude is associated with an increased risk for a first psychotic episode. *Biol Psychiatry* 68 (7):642–48.

Varese, F., Barkus, E., et al. 2012a. Dissociation mediates the relationship between childhood trauma and hallucination-proneness. *Psychol Med* 42 (5):1025–36.

Varese, F., Smeets, F., et al. 2012b. Childhood adversities increase the risk of psychosis: A meta-analysis of patient-control, prospective- and cross-sectional cohort studies. *Schizophr Bull* 38 (4):661–71.

Vazza, G., Bertolin, C., et al. 2007. Genome-wide scan supports the existence of a susceptibility locus for schizophrenia and bipolar disorder on chromosome 15q26. *Mol Psychiatry* 12 (1):87–93.

Warner, R., Laugharne, J., et al. 1999. Retinal function as a marker for cell membrane omega-3 fatty acid depletion in schizophrenia: a pilot study. *Biol Psychiatry* 45 (9):1138–42.

Woodberry, K. A., Giuliano, A. J., et al. 2008. Premorbid IQ in schizophrenia: A meta-analytic review. *Am J Psychiatry* 165 (5):579–87.

Wynn, J. K., Jahshan, C., et al. 2013. Event-related potential examination of facial affect processing in bipolar disorder and schizophrenia. *Psychol Med* 43 (1):109–17.

4

Sleep Schedule, Patterns, and Problems of Children and Adolescents Seen in Child Mental Health Practice

Susan Shur-Fen Gau and Huey-Ling Chiang

Sleep disturbances are frequently experienced by youths with neuropsychiatric disorders and significantly impact the symptom severity of those disorders and aggravate the functional impairment of the patients, the burden on caregivers and the family's quality of life. There is a bi-directional interaction between sleep and psychiatric problems in children and adolescents with neuropsychiatric disorders, so careful consideration is required to understand the nature of the problems and how best to intervene.

Sleep disturbance is a common symptom of depression, bipolar, or anxiety disorders in adult patients, but, given the relatively few studies, the clinical picture is less clear for children and adolescents. However, emerging evidence in recent years indicates that sleep is an important issue in attention-deficit/hyperactivity disorder (ADHD), autism spectrum disorders (ASD), and other childhood neuropsychiatric disorders. This chapter summarizes the sleep schedules, patterns, and problems relevant to the clinical practice of mental health professionals in children and adolescents with ADHD, ASD, and epilepsy. Additionally, the sleep patterns and problems of children and adolescents with depression, anxiety disorders, and bipolar disorder are reviewed but more briefly due to the relatively limited available data from child populations.

ATTENTION-DEFICIT/HYPERACTIVITY DISORDER (ADHD)

Based on parental reports, the prevalence of sleep problems is around 25–50 percent in children with ADHD, consistently higher than that of typically developing (TD) children. Common complaints include difficulties initiating or maintaining sleep, problems waking in the morning, and excessive daytime sleepiness. However, we need to be cautious when interpreting results based on parental reports. First, research using objective measures of sleep, such as polysomnography and actigraphy, did not support the higher risk of several sleep problems reported by parents of children with ADHD. However, objective measures provided other evidence of different sleep architectures and increased risk of sleep apnea and periodic limb movement disorder (PLMD) in children with ADHD (Cortese et al., 2009). Second, the association between ADHD symptoms and sleep problems is complex. Some primary sleep disorders are found to be associated with inattention and hyperactivity, which are often mistaken for ADHD symptoms (Chervin et al., 2002b). Therefore, the importance of a careful ADHD diagnosis based on clinical or structured diagnostic interviews is highlighted (Gau and Chiang, 2009). Third, sleep problems are more common in children with anxiety, depression, oppositional defiant disorder, and other psychiatric conditions, and these psychiatric comorbidities are more likely to develop in children with ADHD. Fourth, psychostimulants, the most commonly used medication for treating ADHD, may prolong sleep onset, reduce sleep efficiency, and shorten sleep duration (Galland et al., 2010). Fifth, the first-night effect, which is the alteration of sleep structure in the sleep laboratory due to unfamiliar environment, should be considered in laboratory-based studies. A first-night effect has been reported in children with ADHD, with a significant increase in wakefulness, reduced sleep efficiency, and prolonged sleep latency compared to the second night (Prihodova et al., 2010). Sixth, developmental trajectories of sleep disturbance should be considered when integrating the results from participants from different age ranges (Scott et al., 2012). Seventh, different subtypes of ADHD, according to DSM-IV, may present different sleep patterns and sleep problems (Chiang et al., 2010). However, relatively few studies have done the subgroup analysis. Therefore, all of these issues need to be considered in assessing sleep problems in youths with ADHD and when interpreting findings regarding the association between ADHD and sleep problems.

Sleep-Onset Difficulty

Sleep-onset difficulty is one of the common sleep problems reported by parents of children with ADHD. In only some of the studies has the ADHD diagnosis been made carefully or the influence of comorbidities and medication status taken into account (Gau and Chiang, 2009; Mayes et al., 2009). Roughly 30 percent of medication-free children with ADHD suffered from chronic sleep-onset insomnia. Although some studies using actigraphy support the differences between children with ADHD and TD children (Hvolby et al., 2008), most objective studies using polysomnography or actigraphy (Owens et al. 2009) did not demonstrate longer sleep-onset latency in children with ADHD. Observer bias is evident in studies using both subjective and objective measures (Hvolby et al., 2008) and both self-reports and parental reports (Owens et al., 2009). Bed-time resistance in children with ADHD and perception of stress in parents may lead to an overestimation of sleep-onset latency by parents (Hvolby et al., 2008). Therefore, the subjective perception of sleep-onset difficulties may be based more on difficulties in managing the problematic behaviors of children with ADHD around bedtime than on an absolute increase in sleep-onset latency (Owens et al., 2009).

Behavioral insomnia, or inappropriate behavior in the context of problematic parent-child interaction, is an important consideration in children with sleep problems. It may present with bedtime resistance, difficulty falling asleep, and/or problems staying asleep, which are associated with poor parenting, parental mental health problems or sleep environment (Corkum et al., 2011). Evaluating sleep problems in the context of parent-child interaction is important. Sleep hygiene education for parents and other behavioral intervention strategies are recommended (see Corkum et al., 2011 for a review). It has been proposed that circadian-rhythm problems with a delayed sleep phase in children with ADHD may partially account for bedtime resistance and sleep-onset difficulties (Van der Heijden et al., 2005), but more evidence is needed to support this viewpoint.

Night-Time Awakening, Sleep Architecture and Sleep Efficiency

Night-time waking is also frequently noted in children with ADHD in both subjective and objective studies (Cortese et al., 2009). Different sleep architecture, higher levels of body and limb movements, and disordered breathing during sleep may accompany frequent night-time awakenings in children with ADHD. Regarding the sleep architecture evaluated by polysomnography, few significant alterations in the macrostructure of sleep, including the percentages of stage 1, stage 2, slow-wave (SWS), and rapid eye movement (REM) sleep, as well as REM sleep latency have been reported (Cortese et al., 2009; Sadeh et al., 2006). Other parameters of polysomnography may show decreased sleep efficiency and increased stage shifts, as reported in several studies of children with ADHD, but there are still many inconsistencies across studies (see Cortese et al., 2009; and Sadeh et al., 2006 for meta-analyses).

Sleep Duration, Sleep Schedule, and Circadian Rhythm Problem

Whether children with ADHD are more likely to have different sleep durations than TD children is still controversial. There have been reports of shorter or longer (Corkum et al., 2001) sleep duration or no difference from TD children (Mayes et al., 2009) by subjective measurements. The inconsistency may be caused by the subjective perception of parents and different interpretations of falling asleep. Most objective studies did not find a difference in total sleep time but revealed an increased intra-individual day-to-day variability in children with ADHD (Hvolby et al., 2008). The intra-individual day-to-day variability of sleep patterns, such as weekday–weekend differences, and unstable circadian rhythm may contribute to the inconsistent findings (Chiang et al., 2010; Gau and Chiang, 2009; Owens et al., 2009).

Although there is generally no difference in bedtime (Gau and Chiang, 2009; Owens et al., 2009), a later rise time on weekdays among children with ADHD has been reported in earlier studies, but this is not supported by recent investigations (Gau and Chiang, 2009; Owens et al., 2009). Greater differences in sleep schedules between weekends and weekdays in subjective studies and a higher intra-individual day-to-day variability using actigraphic monitoring (Hvolby et al., 2008; Owens et al., 2009) may explain the inconsistent findings. Therefore, children with ADHD tend to have an unstable sleep schedule and disturbed circadian rhythm which is not necessarily reflected in the average bedtime and rise time (Owens et al., 2009). Behavioral insomnia still needs to be considered as a cause of unstable sleep schedules in ADHD children, in that inappropriate sleep habits may lead to disturbed sleep schedules (Corkum et al., 2011).

Children with ADHD may have a delayed sleep phase. This reflects a circadian rhythm problem and also the possible cause of sleep-onset difficulty (Van der Heijden et al., 2005). Van der Heijden et al. used salivary melatonin as a marker of circadian phase to survey the possible cause of sleep-onset insomnia. The onset of secretion of melatonin occurred later in ADHD children with insomnia than in ADHD children without insomnia. This implies that the sleep-onset insomnia in ADHD is related to a delayed sleep phase (Van der Heijden et al. 2005).

Parasomnias (Nightmares, Sleep Terrors, Sleep-Talking, Sleepwalking, Enuresis, Bruxism)

Studies concerning parasomnias are mostly focused on periodic limb movement in sleep (PLMS) (e.g., O'Brien et al., 2003) and sleep disordered breathing (SDB) (e.g., Huang et al., 2004), which have been reported more consistently in children with ADHD. However, there is less information about other presentations of parasomnia, which mainly depends on self-reports and is limited by different assessment methods and potential misperception. Parasomnia may be highly prevalent in children with ADHD. According to Silvestri et al. (2009) motor restlessness has been reported in 50 percent of ADHD children, sleep walking in 48 percent, night terrors in 38 percent, and confusional arousals in 29 percent of these children (Silvestri et al., 2009). Some studies report more frequent episodes of enuresis (Mayes et al., 2009; O'Brien et al., 2003), nightmares (Mayes et al., 2009), sleep terrors, bruxism (Gau and Chiang, 2009), sleep-talking, and sleepwalking (Gau and Chiang, 2009; Mayes et al., 2009) in children with ADHD. One study showed a positive association between ADHD and parasomnia as a whole (Owens et al., 2000), but another study failed to demonstrate such an association (Corkam et al., 1999).

Restless Legs Syndrom / Periodic Limb Movement in Sleep (RLS/PLMS)

RLS and PLMS are highly comorbid conditions, and they are the most evidenced sleep disorders in children with ADHD. The prevalence rate of RLS or RLS symptoms may be up to 44 percent in children with ADHD. RLS mimics ADHD symptoms and vice versa, so careful clinical diagnosis is especially important to clarify the relationship between RLS and ADHD. Under a more careful clinical diagnosis the prevalence of RLS is around 25 percent (Silvestri et al., 2009). Several studies support a higher prevalence of RLS in children with ADHD than in controls (Picchietti et al., 1998; Silvestri et al., 2009).

PLMS greater than five times per hour of sleep is also prevalent in children with ADHD, ranging from 10 percent (Huang et al., 2004) to 67 percent (Picchietti et al., 1999) across different studies. Most studies using the standard diagnostic criteria of ADHD supported a higher prevalence of PLMS in children with ADHD (see table 4.1).

Sleep Disordered Breathing (SDB)/Obstructive Sleep Apnea (OSA)

SDB, including OSA, is also one of the frequently studied sleep problems in youths with ADHD. Although some studies report that SDB is

Table 4.1. Studies investigating PLMS/PLMD in children and adolescents with attention-deficit hyperactivity disorder (ADHD)

Study	*Sample size*	*Age*	*Study design*	*Measures/ Assessment of PLMS*	*Major findings*
Prihodova, 2010	57	6–12	Cross-sectional, Clinical-based	Polysomnography	There was no significant difference in PLMS between control and ADHD groups.
Goraya, 2009	33	3–16	Retrospective, Clinical-based	Polysomnography	PLMS were common (30%) among children with ADHD who have symptoms of disturbed sleep.
Sangal, 2005	40	6–14	Cross-sectional, Clinical-based	Polysomnography	No PLMD in ADHD children without snoring plus either observed apneic episodes in sleep or excessive daytime sleepiness, or restless legs at night.
Kirov, 2004	34	8–15	Cross-sectional, Clinical-based	Polysomnography	Total movement time during sleep was not significantly different in ADHD compared with normal control.
Huang, 2004	115	6–12	Cross-sectional, Clinical-based	Polysomnography	Nine (10.2%) of the ADHD group had five or more PLMS per hour, but none in the control group.
Golan, 2004	66	12.4±4.6	Cross-sectional, Clinical-based	Polysomnography	Five (15%) of the ADHD group had PLMS versus none in the control group.
Cooper, 2004	38	4–16	Cross-sectional, Clinical-based	Polysomnography	PLMS in the ADHD group was not different from the control group.

O'Brien, 2003	149	ADHD from clinical/community samples: 8.0±1.6 / 6.6±0.4, Control 6.7±0.4	Cross-sectional, Community and clinical samples	Polysomnography	PLMS with associated arousals was higher in clinical referred ADHD than the other groups, but there were no differences between community ADHD samples and controls.
Crabtree, 2003	142	5–7	Cross-sectional, Community and clinical samples, PLMD with/without ADHD	Polysomnography	Children with PLMD and ADHD had a significantly greater number of arousals associated with PLMS than children with PLMD only
Konofal, 2001	49	5–10	Cross-sectional, Clinical-based	Polysomnography	ADHD children have higher levels of nocturnal activity than controls.
Picchietti, 1999	24	5–12	Cross-sectional, Clinical-based	Polysomnography	The prevalence of PLMS (67%) was higher in the children with ADHD than in the control.
Picchietti, 1998	56	2–15	Cross-sectional, Clinical-based	Polysomnography	The prevalence of PLMS (44%) was higher in the children with ADHD than in the control.

associated with ADHD-related symptoms (Chervin et al., 2002a), an association with the ADHD diagnosis is controversial (Huang et al., 2004; Sadeh et al., 2006). The results of questionnaire-based studies are suggestive of increased snoring (Gau and Chiang, 2009) and SDB (Gruber et al., 2009) in children with ADHD. However, even though some objective studies using polysomnography (Golan et al., 2004; Gruber et al., 2009; Huang et al., 2004) and a meta-analysis (Cortese et al., 2009) revealed such an association, other studies (Cooper et al., 2004; Galland et al., 2011; Kirov et al., 2004; O'Brien et al., 2003) including a meta-analysis failed to show an association (Sadeh et al., 2006) (see table 4.2). Wide variations in the definition of apneas and hypoapneas in children may contribute to this inconsistency in studies using polysomnography.

Daytime Sleepiness

Daytime sleepiness may be the consequence of sleep problems or a delayed sleep phase, or be caused by an intrinsic problem with arousal dysregulation in children with ADHD (Prihodova et al., 2010). Daytime sleepiness can be measured objectively by the Multiple Sleep Latency Test (MSLT). Children with ADHD are sleepier, according to self-reports (Owens et al., 2009), and have an increased number of naps and shorter nap sleep latency as measured by the MSLT (Golan et al., 2004). However, Prihodova and colleagues (2010) found no proof of increased daytime sleepiness in the ADHD group but did find significant vigilance variability during the MSLT (Prihodova et al., 2010).

Sleep and ADHD Subtypes

Due to the heterogeneity of ADHD, the potentially distinctive sleep patterns and sleep problems among ADHD subgroups may confound research findings. One of the widely used subtyping systems is the three subtypes of ADHD according to DSM-IV: predominantly inattentive type (ADHD-I), predominantly hyperactive-impulsive type (ADHD-HI), and combined type (ADHD-C). Since most previous studies have a small ADHD-HI subtype sample (Chiang et al., 2010) or no ADHD-HI subtype sample (Mayes et al., 2009), results regarding the ADHD-HI subtype are rare and less convincing. In addition, since subjective studies have relatively small sample sizes, comparisons among ADHD subtypes are relatively sparse.

Children with different subtypes of ADHD may have specific sleep patterns. Research on this issue is relatively rare, and the results are divergent (Chiang et al., 2010; Mayes et al., 2009; Wiggs et al., 2005). For example, Wiggs et al. (2005) found no subtype differences and earlier bedtime in children with ADHD-I, while Chiang et al. (2010) found earlier

Table 4.2. Studies investigating SDB/OSA in children and adolescents with attention-deficit hyperactivity disorder (ADHD)

Study	*Sample size*	*Age*	*Study design*	*Measures/Assessment of SDB and OSA*	*Major findings*
Galland, 2011	56	6~12	Cross-sectional, Clinical-based	Parent-report, Polysomnography	There was no significant difference in snoring and mild SDB (AHI >1 and <2) between control and ADHD groups.
Prihodova, 2010	57	6~12	Cross-sectional, Clinical-based	Polysomnography	There was no significant difference in SDB between control and ADHD groups.
Goraya, 2009	33	3~16	Retrospective, Clinical-based	Polysomnography	OSA were common (24%) among children with ADHD who have symptoms of disturbed sleep.
Huang, 2007	86	6~12	Cross-sectional, Clinical-based, ADHD children with mild OSA	Polysomnography	Inattention and hyperactivity reduced after treating OSA by adenotonsillectomy or treating ADHD with stimulant.
Sangal, 2005	40	6~14	Cross-sectional, Clinical-based	Polysomnography	No OSA in ADHD children without snoring plus either observed apneic episodes in sleep or excessive daytime sleepiness, or restless legs at night.
Kirov, 2004	34	8~15	Cross-sectional, Clinical-based	Polysomnography	Apnea and hypopnea during sleep was not significantly different in ADHD compared with normal control.
Golan, 2004	66	12.4±4.6	Cross-sectional, Clinical-based	Polysomnography	ADHD children had more signs of SDB (50%), compared the control group.
Huang, 2004	115	6~12	Cross-sectional, Clinical-based	Polysomnography	ADHD children had a higher AHI (56.8% AHI>1, 19.3% AHI>5) than the control children.
Cooper, 2004	38	4~16	Cross-sectional, Clinical-based	Polysomnography	ADHD group is normal in AHI, and had no difference with controls.
O'Brien, 2003	149	ADHD from clinical/ community samples: 8.0±1.6 / 6.6±0.4, Control 6.7±0.4	Cross-sectional, Community and clinical samples	Polysomnography	AHI and apnea index did not differ in the three groups.

bedtimes in children with ADHD-C and ADHD-HI on weekdays. The differences in weekend sleep patterns among subtypes seem less apparent (Chiang et al., 2010). A polysomnography study showed that children with ADHD-I may have better sleep efficiency and less fragmented sleep than children with ADHD-C.

As for daytime sleepiness, children with ADHD-I are most likely to show increased sleepiness as determined by subjective reports (Chiang et al., 2010; Mayes et al., 2009) and MSLT. Children with ADHD-C may also be sleepier than TD children (Chiang et al., 2010), but there is negative evidence from other studies (Mayes et al., 2009). Therefore, the severity of inattentive symptoms may better account for the level of daytime sleepiness between different ADHD subtypes (Chiang et al., 2010).

Children with ADHD-C may have more sleep problems/disorders than those with ADHD-I, with significantly more trouble falling asleep, restlessness during sleep, waking during the night, nightmares (Mayes et al., 2009), and increased movement during sleep. Children with ADHD-C and ADHD-I, but not those with ADHD-HI, tend to have more daytime napping (Chiang et al., 2010). Children with ADHD-C and ADHD-HI are more likely to have RLS and PLMS compared to those with ADHD-I (Silvestri et al., 2009).

Children with ADHD-I, but not those with ADHD-C, tend to have hypersomnia (Chiang et al., 2010). The greater number of sleep problems in children with ADHD-I, as compared with non-ADHD, is supported by one study (Chiang et al., 2010) but not another (Mayes et al., 2009). Chronic nocturnal snoring was more prevalent in children with ADHD-HI in two studies (Chiang et al., 2010), but another study did not demonstrate a difference among subtypes (Wiggs et al., 2005). Other studies showed no subtype differences in dyssomnia, parasomnia, or sleep-disordered breathing (Wiggs et al., 2005).

Consequence of Sleep Problems in ADHD

Both ADHD and sleep problems cause behavioral problems and impaired academic performance, and sleep problems may further exacerbate inattentive and hyperactive symptoms (Chervin et al., 2002b). Screening for other psychiatric comorbidities and the side-effects of medication such as psychostimulants are necessary because both have detrimental effects on sleep (Gau and Chiang, 2009).

AUTISM SPECTRUM DISORDER (ASD)

Sleep problems are common in children with ASD (including autistic disorder [autism], Asperger's disorder, and atypical autism), and approximately 40 percent to 80 percent of these children have at least one frequent sleep problem (Reynolds and Malow 2011). The prevalence of sleep problems in children with ASD is even higher than in children with other developmental disabilities. Although cognitive disability is a risk factor for sleep problems, the association between ASD and sleep problems seems independent from cognitive function in some studies (Krakowiak et al., 2008). Children with high-functioning autism and Asperger's disorder also have a high rate of sleep problems (Paavonen et al., 2008). Controlling for mental retardation as a confounding variable is still suggested because some reports reveal an increased proportion of severely developmentally delayed children with ASD who have sleep problems (Miano et al., 2007). Subanalysis of sleep problems in autism, "pervasive developmental disorders—not otherwise specified" (PDD-NOS), and Asperger's disorder can provide different information as well (Souders et al., 2009). Other psychiatric comorbidities, such as anxiety, depression, and ADHD, which can contribute to or exacerbate sleep problems, also need attention in children with ASD (Malow et al., 2006). Medical comorbidities, such as asthma and epilepsy, also increase the risk of sleep problems in children with ASD. In addition, the presentation of sleep problems may differ in different age groups. Toddlers and young children with ASD report more bedtime resistance, sleep anxiety, parasomnias, and night awakenings, while adolescents with ASD exhibit delayed sleep onset, shorter sleep duration, and daytime sleepiness (Goldman et al., 2012).

Dyssomnia

Sleep-onset insomnia and night awakenings are the most evident and highly prevalent sleep problems in children with ASD (Chou et al., 2012; Krakowiak et al., 2008; Reynolds and Malow, 2011). The majority of these studies are based on parental reports. Questionnaires and sleep diaries completed by parents are more likely to exhibit bedtime resistance (Giannotti et al., 2011), sleep-onset delay (Giannotti et al., 2011; Krakowiak et al., 2008), frequent and prolonged night awakenings (Giannotti et al., 2011; Krakowiak et al., 2008, Souders et al., 2009), early morning waking, shortened sleep duration, and sleep–wake cycle disturbance (Chou et al., 2012). However, parents of children with ASD may slightly over-report sleep problems as a result of their own stress (Goodlin-Jones et al., 2008). Objective studies using actigraphy and polysomnography consistently confirm increased sleep latency, frequent night awakenings, and shorter sleep duration in children with ASD (Goodlin-Jones et al., 2008; Miano et al., 2007).

Behavioral insomnia is also an important manifestation of sleep problems among children with ASD. The maladaptive bedtime routines associated with ASD, which include not understanding the expectations of parents (asking them to go to sleep) and difficulty transitioning from preferred activities to sleep, reflect deficits in communication ability and high insistency (Kotagal and Broomall, 2012).

Sleep Architecture

Studies using polysomography have demonstrated a variety of differences in sleep architecture in children with ASD (Cortesi et al., 2010), including lower sleep efficiency, increased stage 1 sleep and decreased SWS, shorter REM latency (Miano et al., 2007) and lower REM sleep percentage. Cyclic alternating pattern (CAP) is characterized as periodic episodes of aroused EEG activity followed by a period of more quiet sleep. Using CAP analysis, a lower CAP rate associated with SWS sleep alteration has been reported in children with ASD suggesting a low level of arousability during SWS (Miano et al., 2007). Poor sleepers among children with ASD without mental retardation showed prolonged sleep latency and decreased sleep efficiency, but the good sleepers with ASD did not differ from the TD children in sleep architecture (Malow et al., 2006). Children with Asperger's disorder may show only minor differences from those with autism in their sleep architecture; those with Asperger's disorder showed an increased CAP rate in SWS (Bruni et al., 2007). The first-night effect also warrants attention in laboratory-based studies because children with ASD may have a relatively weak ability to adapt to the new sleep environment. The only study focusing on the first-night effect showed fewer minutes of night awakening and increased sleep efficiency on night two, but no change in the following conditions: total sleep time, REM sleep percentage, and REM sleep latency (Buckley et al., 2013). Taken together, a single-night polysomnographic study may be sufficient to provide information about total sleep time and REM parameters in children with ASD.

Autistic regression refers to symptoms of autism becoming apparent after a period of relatively normal development and including the loss of previously acquired skills. This typically occurs between one and three years of age. It has also been proposed that children with regressive autism had less efficient sleep, less total sleep time, prolonged sleep latency, prolonged REM latency, more night awakenings (Giannotti et al., 2011), circadian rhythm problems (delayed sleep, irregular or sleep/wake type phase syndrome), and a lower CAP rate in stage 2 sleep than those without regression (Giannotti et al., 2011).

Parasomnia

Parasomnias need to be distinguished from epileptic seizures, especially as the prevalence of epilepsy is relatively high in children with ASD.

However, little is known about the parasomnias in ASD. Some studies suggest that parasomnias increase in children with ASD (Gail Williams et al., 2004), while others report no increased rate. Questionnaire-based studies report the presence of various parasomnias, such as sleepwalking and bruxism, while others failed to demonstrate different risks of parasomnias, except more nocturnal enuresis in children with ASD (Gail Williams et al., 2004). One study reported only increased bruxism in children with Asperger's disorder (Paavonen et al., 2008).

REM sleep behavior disorder involves abnormal behavior during the REM sleep phase because of the absence of the normal physiologic generalized muscle paralysis. Polysomnography showed a high rate of REM sleep behavior disorder in a case series of children with ASD, but another study did not support the finding (Malow et al., 2006).

RLS/PLMS

PLMS has been suggested to be related to autism, in that 4.8-6.5 percent of children with PLMS meet the diagnosis of ASD. However, no direct evidence has been reported. Research into PLMS in ASD children is difficult to conduct because of the children's low tolerance for polysomnography. Making a diagnosis of RLS is further complicated because of their limited ability to verbally articulate their symptoms (Pullen et al., 2011).

SDB

SDB was found to be associated with ASD in one study (Paavonen et al., 2008) but not in others (Chou et al., 2012; Gail Williams et al., 2004). In a case report, treating OSA by adenotonsillectomy improved daytime behavior in children with ASD. Although SDB is not necessarily more common in ASD, SDB is still prevalent in such children and associated with daytime behavior problems (Chervin et al., 2002a). Considering that ASD and ADHD symptoms are highly comorbid, and SDB is related to ADHD symptoms (Chervin et al., 2002a), SDB is still worth investigating in children with ASD.

Daytime Sleepiness

The prevalence of daytime sleepiness in children with ASD has been reported to be 31 percent to 63 percent (Bruni et al., 2007), and ASD children have more daytime sleepiness (Paavonen et al., 2008) and daytime napping (Chou et al., 2012) than TD children. Comorbid epilepsy, insomnia, and parasomnias are also risk factors for daytime sleepiness (Bruni et al., 2007).

Consequences of Sleep Problems in ASD

Sleep problems may exacerbate autistic symptoms and emotional and behavioral problems in children with ASD (Malow et al., 2006) and especially worsen repetitive behaviors and the need for sameness. Sleep problems in children with ASD correlate with the sleep problems of their parents and unaffected siblings (Chou et al., 2012), and the parents tend to suffer from increased psychological distress, physical complaints, and marital maladjustment .

EPILEPSY

According to a questionnaire-based survey, the prevalence of sleep disturbance among children with epilepsy was estimated to be around 45 percent—significantly higher than that of their siblings and healthy controls (Byars et al., 2008; Wirrell et al., 2005). However, multiple links between epilepsy and sleep need to be clarified. First, epilepsy, especially nocturnal frontal lobe epilepsy, mimics some sleep disorders, such as parasomnias, sleep-related breathing disorders, and sleep-related movement disorders (Kothare and Kaleyias, 2010). Recording episodes with video EEG polysomnography will help the differential diagnosis. Second, several factors may contribute to increased sleep problems in children with epilepsy, including the type of seizure, the origin of the epileptic focus, and seizure frequency. For example, sleep architecture, especially REM sleep, is more preserved during seizure-free nights but disrupted during nights with partial seizures. Patients with temporal lobe epilepsy tend to have sleep disorganization compared to those with extra-temporal foci. Children with refractory epilepsy had more sleep problems than children with better control of seizures (Batista and Nunes, 2007). However, most observations are drawn from studies of adults with epilepsy (see Matos et al., 2010 for a review). Third, the effect of anti-epileptic drugs (AEDs) and other comorbid psychiatric conditions are important confounders when interpreting the association between epilepsy and sleep problems. Medications for epilepsy may impact sleep differently: benzodiazepines, barbiturates, phenytoin, or carbamazepine which have detrimental effects on sleep, while lamotrigine and gabapentin seem to improve sleep stability. Fourth, among children with epilepsy, those comorbid with developmental delay and mental retardation have more sleep problems than those without developmental delay (Batista and Nunes, 2007). On the other hand, sleep fragmentation and deprivation can trigger or exacerbate epilepsy (Matos et al., 2010). Primary sleep disorders, such as OSA, may worsen epilepsy and treatment of these sleep disorders improves seizure control. Therefore, sleep problems can be present in children with epilepsy contributing to sleep fragmentation, which in turn leads to difficulty controlling epilepsy (Matos et al., 2010). Children with epilepsy need careful evaluation to determine whether sleep affects epilepsy or epilepsy modifies sleep.

Sleep Pattern

No apparent differences have been reported in bedtime, rising time, and total sleep duration at night between children with epilepsy, their siblings, or healthy controls. One polysomnographic study revealed decreased total bed time and total sleep time in children with partial refractory epilepsy (Nunes et al., 2003).

Dyssomnia

Children with epilepsy tend to have more bedtime resistance, sleep onset delay, and night awakening than their siblings (Byars et al., 2008) and healthy controls (Batista and Nunes, 2007), according to questionnaire-based studies reported by their parents. Among children with epilepsy, those with predominantly nocturnal seizures, poor control of seizures (refractory epilepsy), and generalized seizures have more sleep problems than their counterparts (Batista and Nunes, 2007).

Sleep Architecture

Instability of REM sleep is most frequently reported in children with epilepsy. Decreased or increased (Kaleyias et al., 2008) REM percentage, increased REM latency, lower sleep efficiency and a higher arousal index (Kaleyias et al., 2008) have been reported in epilepsy. In addition, children with poor seizure control had a significantly more disturbed microstructure of sleep than children who were seizure-free or children with good seizure control (Kaleyias et al., 2008). Although a reduced amount of REM sleep has been seen after both daytime and nocturnal epilepsy, only nocturnal epilepsy significantly reduced sleep efficiency and increased REM latency. However, other studies did not support nocturnal epilepsy as a risk factor for more disrupted sleep architecture. The characteristics of epilepsy among study participants and chronic use of different AEDs among study participants may partially explain the inconsistency among studies.

Parasomnia

Studies report a 63 percent incidence of restless sleep, 67 percent incidence of snoring (Becker et al. 2004), and 53 percent incidence of parasomnia (Maganti et al., 2006) in children with epilepsy. These children have more parasomnias than their siblings (Byars et al., 2008) and healthy controls (Batista and Nunes, 2007; Becker et al., 2004).

Epilepsy can occur at any stage of non-REM sleep but more commonly during lighter stages than deep sleep and rarely during REM sleep. However, non-REM parasomnias, such as sleepwalking, sleep terrors, and confusional arousal, can be difficult to differentiate from nocturnal frontal lobe epilepsy. Use of the frontal lobe epilepsy and parasomnia scale, a validated questionnaire for nocturnal events, and video-EEG-polysomnography can help reach an accurate diagnosis (see Derry, 2012 for a review).

RLS/PLMS

There has been no study on RLS, and few studies on PLMS in children with epilepsy. PLMS was reported to have occurred in four (10 percent) participants in one study of forty children with epilepsy (Kaleyias et al., 2008), but other studies did not support a difference from non-epileptic controls (Becker et al., 2004).

SDB/OSA

OSA is the most well-studied sleep disorder in adults with epilepsy, but studies of children are relatively scarce. These studies of child populations contain relatively small numbers of patients. Children with epilepsy have a high prevalence of OSA, ranging from 30 percent to 65 percent (Maganti et al., 2006). Furthermore, 80 percent of children with epilepsy and sleep complaints referred for polysomnographic study were identified as having OSA (Becker et al., 2004). In a study of children with epilepsy based on questionnaires, a higher risk of OSA was related to refractory epilepsy and taking more than one AED, but was not associated with type of seizures.

Although controlling epilepsy with medication is important, some AEDs may cause weight gain, and benzodiazepines may reduce respiratory drive and upper airway tone, which may aggravate the conditions of OSA and its impact on epilepsy. OSA may also cause sleep deprivation, which may have a detrimental effect on seizure control among children with epilepsy. Improvement in seizure control can be noted after treatment of concomitant OSA (Segal et al., 2012). Therefore, identification and treatment of both epilepsy and OSA is important to optimize treatment outcome.

Daytime Sleepiness

Excessive daytime sleepiness is very common in children with epilepsy compared to their siblings (Byars et al., 2008) and healthy controls (Batista and Nunes, 2007). A daytime sleepiness prevalence rate of 63 percent (Becker et al., 2004) to 76 percent (Maganti et al., 2006) has been reported by parents, and 46 percent in self-reports (Maganti et al., 2006). Sleep problems, such as SDB and parasomnias are important factors for daytime sleepiness, but the level of daytime sleepiness did not differ between children with generalized and localization-related epilepsy (Maganti et al., 2006). AEDs may cause daytime sleepiness and changes in sleep architecture, and disturbance in sleep architecture may also predispose to daytime sleepiness.

Influences of Sleep Problems in Epilepsy

Sleep disturbances and excessive daytime sleepiness are known to have negative effects on emotional and behavioral problems, neuropsychological functioning, social functioning, and quality of life (Byars et al., 2008). Concurrent treatment of these two conditions in children with epilepsy is recommended, and improvement in seizure control and daily functioning can be expected (Segal et al., 2012).

OTHER PSYCHIATRIC DISORDERS OF CHILDHOOD AND ADOLESCENCE

Depression

Sleep disturbance, either insomnia or hypersomnia, are symptoms of depression according to diagnostic criteria. Subjective sleep disturbance is a frequent complaint in children with depression: 54 percent complained of insomnia alone, 9 percent complained of hypersomnia alone, and 10 percent had both disturbances during a depressive episode (Liu et al., 2007). They also report poor sleep quality, increased number of awakenings, more night-waking, circadian disturbance, and daytime sleepiness (Bertocci et al., 2005; Dahl et al., 1996). However, sleep disturbance reported subjectively by depressed children may reflect a biased perception. Some polysomnographic studies have failed to find objective evidence of sleep disturbance in children with depression, although subjective sleep complaints were reported at the same time (Bertocci et al., 2005). Children and adolescents with depression may have prolonged sleep latency and reduced REM latency in polysomnographic studies (Dahl et al., 1996).

Studies of adolescents with depression have reported stronger evidence of objective sleep disturbances than studies of children.

Effect of Antidepressants on Sleep

Most antidepressant drugs have been shown to impact sleep architecture. The antidepressants most commonly prescribed for children, selective serotonin-reuptake inhibitors, are associated with increased sleep latency, increased REM latency, increased night awakenings, and decreased REM sleep.

Cross-sectional studies have shown that sleep disturbance is associated with the severity of depression and suicidal risk in patients with depression. During a depressive episode, sleep-disturbed children and adolescents had more depressive symptoms and greater severity of depression than those without sleep disturbance (Liu et al., 2007). In addition, sleep disturbance is associated with increased risk of completed suicide in depressed adolescents in analyses accounting for the severity of depressive symptoms (Goldstein et al., 2008). Longitudinal studies reveal that sleep problems increase vulnerability to depression in children, and that sleep problems at age eight predicted depression at age ten, but the converse was not found (Gregory et al., 2009).

Bipolar Disorder

Sleep disturbance is a core symptom of bipolar disorder. Children with bipolar disorder may present with insomnia or hypersomnia during depressive states and a decreased need for sleep during manic or hypomanic states. Sleep disturbance, insomnia or parasomnias, may be one of the important antecedents or early signs of bipolar disorder in children, according to parent reports. Around 95 percent of children with bipolar disorder exhibited sleep disturbance, including insomnia and parasomnias, and 45 percent of them had sleep disturbance as an initial symptom (Faedda et al., 2004). More resistance to going to sleep, difficulty initiating sleep, restless sleep, nightmares (Mehl et al., 2006), and a reduced need for sleep (Holtmann et al., 2007) via subjective reports have been specifically mentioned compared to healthy controls (Mehl et al., 2006), ADHD patients (Geller et al., 2002), and clinical controls with comparable levels of psychopathology other than bipolar disorder (Holtmann et al., 2007).

Few studies used objective measures to investigate the sleep architecture of children with bipolar disorder have been carried out. Decreased sleep efficiency, increased night awakening, increased slow wave sleep, and reduced REM sleep were among the common sleep architecture problems in children with bipolar disorder (Mehl et al., 2006). The sleep architecture recorded during the depressive state differed in adolescents with unipolar and bipolar disorder, in that the bipolar group had more stage 1 sleep, increased REM latency, lower REM density, and reduced REM sleep compared to the unipolar group.

High rates of psychiatric comorbidity, such as anxiety, ADHD, and oppositional defiant disorder (Faedda et al., 2004), which are also associated with increased sleep disturbance, are reported in children and adolescents with bipolar disorder. In addition, medications used to treat bipolar disorder may contribute to more sleep disturbance (Harvey et al., 2009). Sleep problems may exacerbate the adverse consequences of bipolar disorder, including deteriorated affect regulation, cognitive functions and quality of life, and also increase the risk of relapse of bipolar disorder (Harvey et al., 2009).

Anxiety Disorder

Sleep disturbance is frequently reported in children with anxiety disorders, with a prevalence rate of 88–90 percent of at least one sleep problem (Chase and Pincus, 2011). Most of these children had multiple sleep disturbances. Among youth with generalized anxiety disorder, 56 percent of children and 49 percent of adolescents experienced a sleep disturbance based on combined parent and child reports. The most common sleep-related problems were insomnia, resistance to sleep alone, and nightmares (Chase and Pincus, 2011). Children with more psychiatric diagnoses or multiple anxiety disorders had an added risk of sleep-related problems (Chase and Pincus, 2011). Sleep-related problems were also positively associated with anxiety severity and interference in daytime functioning. A longitudinal study using a large community sample suggested that sleep problems in early childhood could predict anxiety disorder more than twenty years later (Gregory et al., 2005).

A polysomnography study revealed children with anxiety disorders had more awakenings and decreased slow-wave sleep than children with depression and more decreased slow-wave sleep than healthy children (Forbes et al., 2008). Another study focusing on children with generalized anxiety disorder exhibited significantly increased sleep onset latency and reduced latency to REM sleep compared to controls (Alfano et al., 2012).

Difficulty falling or staying asleep (increased arousal) and nightmares (reexperiencing) are common symptoms of post-traumatic stress disorder (PTSD). Children exposed to trauma or diagnosed with PTSD have significantly more sleep disturbances than non-trauma-exposed controls. Commonly reported sleep disturbances include difficulty falling asleep, difficulty maintaining sleep, nightmares, and bedwetting (Kovachy et al.,

2013). However, most studies are questionnaire-based without objective measures.

Among anxiety disorders, sleep disturbance has been less linked to obsessive-compulsive disorder (OCD) in clinical practice, but it has been reported that up to 92 percent of children with OCD had sleep problems. Sleep problems were positively associated with OCD symptom severity and other emotional problems (Storch et al., 2008).

Although there is a high prevalence of sleep disturbance in children with anxiety disorder, studies are relatively rare. Comorbid depression and use of medications may be the most important confounding factors that need to be addressed in future research.

CONCLUSION

Given the high prevalence of sleep problems associated with neuropsychiatric conditions, pediatric health care practitioners are recommended to assess sleep schedules, patterns and problems in children and adolescents with neuropsychiatric disorders. Screening for other psychiatric comorbidities and the side effects of medications is also necessary because both have adverse effects on sleep. In addition to managing the symptoms of neuropsychiatric disorders, it is important to screen, diagnose, and treat sleep disturbances in these children. The research implications are as follows: first, the specificity of the associations between neuropsychiatric disorder and sleep disturbance warrants further clarification. Second, the potential confounding effects of other neuropsychiatric comorbidities and use of medication need to be considered when analyzing the association between sleep disturbance and the disorders reviewed herein. Finally, further investigation combining subjective (such as parental reports, self-reports, interviews, etc.) and objective (such as polysomnography, actigraphy, MSLT, etc.) measures with a longitudinal design is encouraged.

REFERENCES

Alfano, C. A., Reynolds, K., Scott, N., Dahl, R. E. & Mellman, T. A. (2012). Polysomnographic sleep patterns of non-depressed, non-medicated children with generalized anxiety disorder. *Journal of Affective Disorders,* doi: 10.1016/j.jad.2012.08.015.

Batista, B. H. & Nunes, M. L. (2007). Evaluation of sleep habits in children with epilepsy. *Epilepsy & Behavior* 11, 60–64.

Becker, D. A., Fennell, E. B. & Carney, P. R. (2004). Daytime behavior and sleep disturbance in childhood epilepsy. *Epilepsy & Behavior* 5, 708–15.

Bertocci, M. A., Dahl, R. E., Williamson, D. E., Iosif, A. M., Birmaher, B., et al. (2005). Subjective sleep complaints in pediatric depression: A controlled study and comparison with EEG measures of sleep and waking. *Journal of American Academy of Child and Adolescent Psychiatry* 44, 1158–66.

Bruni, O., Ferri, R., Vittori, E., Novelli, L., Vignati, M., et al. (2007). Sleep architecture and NREM alterations in children and adolescents with Asperger syndrome. *Sleep* 30, 1577–85.

Buckley, A., Wingert, K., Swedo, S., Thurm, A., Sato, S., et al. (2013). First night effect analysis in a cohort of young children with autism spectrum disorder. *Journal of Clinical Sleep Medicine* 9, 67–70.

Byars, A. W., Byars, K. C., Johnson, C. S., DeGrauw, T. J., Fastenau, P. S., et al. (2008). The relationship between sleep problems and neuropsychological functioning in children with first recognized seizures. *Epilepsy & Behavior* 13, 607–13.

Chase, R. M. & Pincus, D. B. (2011). Sleep-related problems in children and adolescents with anxiety disorders. *Behavioral Sleep Medicine* 9, 224–36.

Chervin, R. D., Archbold, K. H., Dillon, J. E., Panahi, P., Pituch, K. J., et al. (2002a). Inattention, hyperactivity, and symptoms of sleep-disordered breathing. *Pediatrics,* 109, 449–56.

Chervin, R. D., Archbold, K. H., Dillon, J. E., Panahi, P., Pituch, K. J., et al. (2002b). Associations between symptoms of inattention, hyperactivity, restless legs, and periodic leg movements. *Sleep* 25, 213–18.

Chiang, H. L., Gau, S. S., Ni, H. C., Chiu, Y. N., Shang, C. Y., et al. (2010). Association between symptoms and subtypes of attention-deficit hyperactivity disorder and sleep problems/disorders. *Journal of Sleep Research* 19, 535–45.

Chou, M. C., Chou, W. J., Chiang, H. L., Wu, Y. Y., Lee, J. C., et al. (2012). Sleep problems among Taiwanese children with autism, their siblings and typically developing children. *Research in Autism Spectrum Disorders* 6, 665–72.

Cooper, J., Tyler, L., Wallace, I. & Burgess, K. R. (2004). No evidence of sleep apnea in children with attention deficit hyperactivity disorder. *Clinical Pediatrics* 43, 609–14.

Corkum, P., Davidson, F. & Macpherson, M. (2011). A framework for the assessment and treatment of sleep problems in children with attention-deficit/hyperactivity disorder. *Pediatric Clinics of North America* 58, 667–83.

Corkum, P., Tannock, R., Moldofsky, H., Hogg-Johnson, S. & Humphries, T. (2001). Actigraphy and parental ratings of sleep in children with attention-deficit/hyperactivity disorder (ADHD). *Sleep* 24, 303–12.

Corkum, P., Moldofsky, H., Hogg-Johnson, S., Humphries, T. & Tannock, R. (1999). Sleep problems in children with attention-deficit/hyperactivity disorder: Impact of subtype, comorbidity, and stimulant medication. *Journal of the American Academy of Child & Adolesant Psychiatry* 38, 1285–93.

Cortese, S., Faraone, S. V., Konofal, E. & Lecendreux, M. (2009). Sleep in children with attention-deficit/hyperactivity disorder: meta-analysis of subjective and objective studies. *Journal of the American Academy of Child & Adolescent Psychiatry* 48, 894–908.

Cortesi, F., Giannotti, F., Ivanenko, A. & Johnson, K. (2010). Sleep in children with autistic spectrum disorder. *Sleep Medicine* 11, 659–64.

Crabtree, V. M., Ivanenko, A., & Gozal, D. (2003). Clinical and parental assessment of sleep in children with attention-deficit/hyperactivity disorder referred to a pediatric sleep medicine center. *Clinical pediatrics* 42, 807–813.

Dahl, R. E., Ryan, N. D., Matty, M. K., Birmaher, B., al-Shabbout, M., et al. (1996). Sleep onset abnormalities in depressed adolescents. *Biological Psychiatry* 39, 400–410.

Derry, C. (2012). Nocturnal Frontal Lobe Epilepsy vs Parasomnias. *Current Treatment Options in Neurology* 14, 451–63.

Faedda, G. L., Baldessarini, R. J., Glovinsky, I. P. & Austin, N. B. (2004). Pediatric bipolar disorder: phenomenology and course of illness. *Bipolar Disorder* 6, 305–13.

Forbes, E. E., Bertocci, M. A., Gregory, A. M., Ryan, N. D., Axelson, D. A., et al. (2008). Objective sleep in pediatric anxiety disorders and major depressive disorder. *Journal of the American Academy of Child & Adolescent Psychiatry* 47, 148–55.

Gail Williams, P., Sears, L. L. & Allard, A. (2004). Sleep problems in children with autism. *Journal of Sleep Research* 13, 265–68.

Galland, B. C., Tripp, E. G., Gray, A. & Taylor, B. J. (2011). Apnea-hypopnea indices and snoring in children diagnosed with ADHD: A matched case-control study. *Sleep and Breathing* 15, 455–62.

Galland, B. C., Tripp, E. G. & Taylor, B. J. (2010). The sleep of children with attention deficit hyperactivity disorder on and off methylphenidate: A matched case-control study. *Journal of Sleep Research* 19, 366–73.

Gau, S. S. & Chiang, H. L. (2009). Sleep problems and disorders among adolescents with persistent and sub-threshold attention-deficit/hyperactivity disorders. *Sleep* 32, 671–79.

Geller, B., Zimerman, B., Williams, M., Delbello, M. P., Frazier, J. & Beringer, L. (2002). Phenomenology of prepubertal and early adolescent bipolar disorder: Examples of elated mood, grandiose behaviors, decreased need for sleep, racing thoughts and hypersexuality. *Journal of Child and Adolescent Psychopharmacology* 12, 3–9.

Giannotti, F., Cortesi, F., Cerquiglini, A., Vagnoni, C. & Valente, D. (2011). Sleep in children with autism with and without autistic regression. *Journal of Sleep Research* 20, 338–47.

Golan, N., Shahar, E., Ravid, S. & Pillar, G. (2004). Sleep disorders and daytime sleepiness in children with attention-deficit/hyperactive disorder. *Sleep* 27, 261–66.

Goldman, S. E., Richdale, A. L., Clemons, T. & Malow, B. A. (2012). Parental sleep concerns in autism spectrum disorders: Variations from childhood to adolescence. *Journal of Autism and Developmental disorders* 42, 531–38.

Goldstein, T. R., Bridge, J. A. & Brent, D. A. (2008). Sleep disturbance preceding completed suicide in adolescents. *Journal of Consulting and Clinical Psychology* 76, 84–91.

Goodlin-Jones, B. L., Tang, K., Liu, J. & Anders, T. F. (2008). Sleep patterns in preschool-age children with autism, developmental delay, and typical development. *Journal of the American Academy of Child & Adolescent Psychiatry* 47, 930–38.

Goraya, J. S., Cruz, M., Valencia, I., Kaleyias, J., Khurana, D. S., Hardison, H. H., Marks, H., Legido, A., & Kothare, S. V. (2009). Sleep study abnormalities in children with attention deficit hyperactivity disorder. *Pediatric neurology* 40, 42–46.

Gregory, A. M., Caspi, A., Eley, T. C., Moffitt, T. E., Oconnor, T. G. & Poulton, R. (2005). Prospective longitudinal associations between persistent sleep problems in childhood and anxiety and depression disorders in adulthood. *Journal of Abnormal Child Psychology* 33, 157–63.

Gregory, A. M., Rijsdijk, F. V., Lau, J. Y., Dahl, R. E. & Eley, T. C. (2009). The direction of longitudinal associations between sleep problems and depression symptoms: a study of twins aged 8 and 10 years. *Sleep* 32, 189–99.

Gruber, R., Xi, T., Frenette, S., Robert, M., Vannasinh, P., et al. (2009). Sleep disturbances in prepubertal children with attention deficit hyperactivity disorder: a home polysomnography study. *Sleep* 32, 343–50.

Harvey, A. G., Talbot, L. S. & Gershon, A. (2009). Sleep disturbance in bipolar disorder across the lifespan. *Clinical Psychology (New York)* 16, 256–77.

Holtmann, M., Bolte, S., Goth, K., Dopfner, M., Pluck, J., et al. (2007). Prevalence of the child behavior checklist-pediatric bipolar disorder phenotype in a German general population sample. *Bipolar Disorder* 9, 895–900.

Huang, Y. S., Chen, N. H., Li, H. Y., Wu, Y. Y., Chao, C. C. & Guilleminault, C. (2004). Sleep disorders in Taiwanese children with attention deficit/hyperactivity disorder. *Journal of Sleep Research* 13, 269–77.

Huang, Y. S., Guilleminault, C., Li, H. Y., Yang, C. M., Wu, Y. Y., & Chen, N. H. (2007). Attention-deficit/hyperactivity disorder with obstructive sleep apnea: A treatment outcome study. *Sleep Medicine* 8, 18–30.

Hvolby, A., Jorgensen, J. & Bilenberg, N. (2008). Actigraphic and parental reports of sleep difficulties in children with attention-deficit/hyperactivity disorder. *Archives of Pediatrics & Adolescent Medicine* 162, 323–29.

Kaleyias, J., Cruz, M., Goraya, J. S., Valencia, I., Khurana, D. S., et al. (2008). Spectrum of polysomnographic abnormalities in children with epilepsy. *Pediatric Neurology* 39, 170–76.

Kirov, R., Kinkelbur, J., Heipke, S., Kostanecka-Endress, T., Westhoff, M., et al. (2004). Is there a specific polysomnographic sleep pattern in children with attention deficit/hyperactivity disorder? *Journal of Sleep Research* 13, 87–93.

Konofal, E., Lecendreux, M., Bouvard, M. P., & Mouren-Simeoni, M. C. (2001). High levels of nocturnal activity in children with attention-deficit hyperactivity disorder: A video analysis. *Psychiatry & Clinical Neurosciences* 55, 97–103.

Kotagal, S. & Broomall, E. (2012). Sleep in children with autism spectrum disorder. *Pediatric Neurology* 47, 242–51.

Kothare, S. V. & Kaleyias, J. (2010). Sleep and epilepsy in children and adolescents. *Sleep Medicine* 11, 674–85.

Kovachy, B., O'Hara, R., Hawkins, N., Gershon, A., Primeau, M. M., Madej, J., & Carrion, V. (2013). Sleep disturbance in pediatric PTSD: Current findings and future directions. *Journal of clinical sleep medicine* 9, 501–10.

Krakowiak, P., Goodlin-Jones, B., Hertz-Picciotto, I., Croen, L. A. & Hansen, R. L. (2008). Sleep problems in children with autism spectrum disorders, developmental delays, and typical development: A population-based study. *Journal of Sleep Research* 17, 197–206.

Liu, X., Buysse, D. J., Gentzler, A. L., Kiss, E., Mayer, L., et al. (2007). Insomnia and hypersomnia associated with depressive phenomenology and comorbidity in childhood depression. *Sleep* 30, 83–90.

Maganti, R., Hausman, N., Koehn, M., Sandok, E., Glurich, I. & Mukesh, B. N. (2006). Excessive daytime sleepiness and sleep complaints among children with epilepsy. *Epilepsy & Behavior* 8, 272–77.

Malow, B. A., Marzec, M. L., McGrew, S. G., Wang, L., Henderson, L. M. & Stone, W. L. (2006). Characterizing sleep in children with autism spectrum disorders: A multidimensional approach. *Sleep* 29, 1563–71.

Matos, G., Andersen, M. L., do Valle, A. C. & Tufik, S. (2010). The relationship between sleep and epilepsy: Evidence from clinical trials and animal models. *Journal of the Neurological Sciences* 295, 1–7.

Mayes, S. D., Calhoun, S. L., Bixler, E. O., Vgontzas, A. N., Mahr, F., et al. (2009). ADHD subtypes and comorbid anxiety, depression, and oppositional-defiant disorder: Differences in sleep problems. *Journal of Pediatric Psychology* 34, 328–37.

Mehl, R. C., O'Brien, L. M., Jones, J. H., Dreisbach, J. K., Mervis, C. B. & Gozal, D. (2006). Correlates of sleep and pediatric bipolar disorder. *Sleep* 29, 193–97.

Miano, S., Bruni, O., Elia, M., Trovato, A., Smerieri, A., et al. (2007). Sleep in children with autistic spectrum disorder: A questionnaire and polysomnographic study. *Sleep Medicine* 9, 64–70.

Nunes, M. L., Ferri, R., Arzimanoglou, A., Curzi, L., Appel, C. C. & Costa da Costa, J. (2003). Sleep organization in children with partial refractory epilepsy. *Journal of Child Neurology* 18, 763–66.

O'Brien, L. M., Ivanenko, A., Crabtree, V. M., Holbrook, C. R., Bruner, J. L., et al. (2003). Sleep disturbances in children with attention deficit hyperactivity disorder. *Pediatric Research* 54, 237–43.

Owens, J., Sangal, R. B., Sutton, V. K., Bakken, R., Allen, A. J. & Kelsey, D. (2009). Subjective and objective measures of sleep in children with attention-deficit/hyperactivity disorder. *Sleep Medicine* 10, 446–56.

Owens, J. A., Maxim, R., Nobile, C., McGuinn, M. & Msall, M. (2000). Parental and self-report of sleep in children with attention-deficit/hyperactivity disorder. *Archives of Pediatrics & Adolescent Medicine* 154, 549–55.

Paavonen, E. J., Vehkalahti, K., Vanhala, R., von Wendt, L., Nieminen-von Wendt, T. & Aronen, E. T. (2008). Sleep in children with Asperger syndrome. *Journal of Autism and Developmental Disorders* 38, 41–51.

Picchietti, D. L., England, S. J., Walters, A. S., Willis, K. & Verrico, T. (1998). Periodic limb movement disorder and restless legs syndrome in children with attention-deficit hyperactivity disorder. *Journal of Child Neurology* 13, 588–94.

Picchietti, D. L., Underwood, D. J., Farris, W. A., Walters, A. S., Shah, M. M., et al. (1999). Further studies on periodic limb movement disorder and restless legs syndrome in children with attention-deficit hyperactivity disorder. *Movement Disorders* 14, 1000–1007.

Prihodova, I., Paclt, I., Kemlink, D., Skibova, J., Ptacek, R. & Nevsimalova, S. (2010). Sleep disorders and daytime sleepiness in children with attention-deficit/hyperactivity disorder: A two-night polysomnographic study with a multiple sleep latency test. *Sleep Medicien* 11, 922–28.

Pullen, S. J., Wall, C. A., Angstman, E. R., Munitz, G. E. & Kotagal, S. (2011). Psychiatric comorbidity in children and adolescents with restless legs syndrome: A retrospective study. *Journal of Clinical Sleep Medicine* 7, 587–96.

Reynolds, A. M. & Malow, B. A. (2011). Sleep and autism spectrum disorders. *Pediatric Clinics of North America* 58, 685–98.

Sadeh, A., Pergamin, L. & Bar-Haim, Y. (2006). Sleep in children with attention-deficit hyperactivity disorder: A meta-analysis of polysomnographic studies. *Sleep Medicine Reviews* 10, 381–98.

Sangal, R. B., Owens, J. A., & Sangal, J. (2005). Patients with attention-deficit/hyperactivity disorder without observed apneic episodes in sleep or daytime sleepiness have normal sleep on polysomnography. *Sleep* 28, 1143–1148.

Scott, N., Blair, P. S., Emond, A. M., Fleming, P. J., Humphreys, J. S., et al. (2012). Sleep patterns in children with ADHD: A population-based cohort study from birth to 11 years. *Journal of Sleep Research, doi: 10.1111/j.1365-2869.2012.01054.x.*

Segal, E., Vendrame, M., Gregas, M., Loddenkemper, T. & Kothare, S. V. (2012). Effect of treatment of obstructive sleep apnea on seizure outcomes in children with epilepsy. *Pediatric Neurology* 46, 359–62.

Silvestri, R., Gagliano, A., Arico, I., Calarese, T., Cedro, C., et al. (2009). Sleep disorders in children with Attention-Deficit/Hyperactivity Disorder (ADHD) recorded overnight by video-polysomnography. *Sleep Medicine* 10, 1132–38.

Souders, M. C., Mason, T. B., Valladares, O., Bucan, M., Levy, S. E., et al. (2009). Sleep behaviors and sleep quality in children with autism spectrum disorders. *Sleep* 32, 1566–78.

Storch, E. A., Murphy, T. K., Lack, C. W., Geffken, G. R., Jacob, M. L. & Goodman, W. K. (2008). Sleep-related problems in pediatric obsessive-compulsive disorder. *Journal of Anxiety Disorders* 22, 877–85.

Van der Heijden, K. B., Smits, M. G., Van Someren, E. J. & Gunning, W. B. (2005). Idiopathic chronic sleep onset insomnia in attention-deficit/hyperactivity disorder: A circadian rhythm sleep disorder. *Chronobiology International* 22, 559–70.

Wiggs, L., Montgomery, P. & Stores, G. (2005). Actigraphic and parent reports of sleep patterns and sleep disorders in children with subtypes of attention-deficit hyperactivity disorder. *Sleep* 28, 1437–45.

Wirrell, E., Blackman, M., Barlow, K., Mah, J. & Hamiwka, L. (2005). Sleep disturbances in children with epilepsy compared with their nearest-aged siblings. *Developmental Medicine & Child Neurology* 47, 754–59.

III

INTERVENTIONS AND PRACTICE

5

Child and Adolescent Mental Health Services in Low- and Middle-Income Countries

The Role of Task Shifting

Marguerite Marlow and Mark Tomlinson

Failing to address the mental health of children and adolescents leads to problems with lifelong consequences (WHO, 2003). The mental health of children and adolescents has received low priority in comparison with their survival and physical health needs. Many mental disorders have their onset during adolescence; however, diagnosis and treatment are often delayed. Failing to intervene in early developmental stages makes it likely that problems will persist, since many adult mental health problems originate early in life (Kessler et al., 2007). For those affected, the severe lack of human resources for health and the inaccessibility of appropriate health services result in significant barriers for care and treatment. Low- and middle-income countries (LAMIC) face a number of challenges in bridging the gap to reach those in need, not least of which is the number of children living out of reach of formal health services and clinics. Extending the reach of health services into communities is crucial to meeting the needs of families in LAMIC.

The implementation of effective interventions for child and adolescent mental health (CAMH) often necessitates a multi-disciplinary team. In

LAMIC, service provision is often not organized in a way that enables effective collaboration between various service platforms, where specialists or multidisciplinary teams rarely exist. Relying on mental health professionals or specialist workers to deliver psychological treatments will only address the needs of a very small proportion of children and adolescents. Strategically delegating responsibilities from specialists to other cadres presents a valuable strategy to address shortages of personnel, the need for scaling up of interventions, and to ensure effectiveness and reach.

"NO HEALTH WITHOUT MENTAL HEALTH"

The UN's Millennium Development Goals (MDGs) is a strategy aimed at addressing global inequalities in the provision of care. With significant gains in mortality and morbidity in many LAMIC, attention has shifted to ensuring that children meet their developmental potential (Grantham-McGregor et al., 2007; Rahman, Mubbashar, Harrington & Gater, 2000). The physical and mental health of children is inextricably linked, making a focus on mental health essential for reducing the burden of illness for children and adolescents (Kieling et al., 2011). More than 75 percent of those presenting with significant anxiety, mood, impulse control, or substance use disorders in the World Mental Health surveys in LAMIC did not receive any preventative care or treatment. In Sub-Saharan Africa, over 90 percent of people living with schizophrenia and other psychoses remain untreated (Patel, Boyce, Collins, Saxena & Horton, 2011a). This is known as the "treatment gap." The situation is worse for CAMH. The WHO Atlas project on child and adolescent mental health resources estimated that up to 20 percent of children and adolescents suffer from mental illness but that only a small minority of these individuals receive the necessary care (WHO, 2005a). Between one-half and two-thirds of all mental health needs of children and adolescents are going unmet in most countries, with significantly higher proportions in LAMIC (WHO, 2005a). The higher proportion of children and adolescents in LAMIC makes the burden greater (Patel, Flisher, Nikapota & Malhotra, 2008). There is also a significant research gap with less than 1 percent of trials addressing the needs of children and adolescents in LAMIC (Klasen & Crombag, 2013; Patel et al., 2007).

Trained child and adolescent mental health specialists (where they exist) are usually located in urban areas and in countries such as South Africa often work privately, further marginalizing peri-urban and rural areas (Eisenberg & Belfer, 2009). There is an urgent need to close the "treatment gap" and to focus on a life-course approach that focuses on CAMH (Collins et al., 2011). Meeting this challenge requires collaboration between various sectors to develop new models of intervention, but it also requires investing in alternative models such as community health workers to deliver services (Tomlinson et al., 2011).

"CARE FROM WITHIN THE HOUSEHOLD, ALL THE WAY TO THE HEALTH FACILITY"

The mental health problems of children and adolescents present specific challenges together with specific risk factors depending on the development stage (Kieling et al., 2011; Patel et al., 2008). In the context of high levels of under-five mortality and morbidity, children at this age often require significant contact with the general health system. In the context of scarce resources that characterize most LAMIC, prevention and promotion interventions are rare and are seen as less important than ensuring survival and adequate physical health. An effective system of care for CAMH must include a continuum of interventions arranged according to the child's and the family's needs (WHO, 2003). Ideally, these should be addressed through a variety of platforms, allowing collaboration between different cadres of health care. Sanders suggests that "this care should be taking place from within the household, at the wider community level, all the way to the health facility" (Sanders, 2010, p. 9). A multi-level approach in the context of the interrelatedness of factors associated with CAMH is essential.

ACCESS TO MENTAL HEALTH CARE: POSSIBLE PLATFORMS FOR PREVENTION AND INTERVENTION

In many countries, child and adolescent mental health services are seen as a subset of general mental health services or child health services. In the context of scarce resources, an important question is to what extent alternative platforms can be utilized to address CAMH needs. Although decentralization of mental health services and integration into the primary health sector is important to improve accessibility and reach, most children with mental health problems are unlikely to access these services. They will in all likelihood first be seen within the education, social service or juvenile justice systems (Burns et al, 1995). In addition, stigmatization and lack of awareness of mental illness may prevent many families from seeking help. Therefore, a family-focused approach to treating problems through community- and home-based interventions is crucial for scale-up of services (Tomlinson, 2010). Delegating curative, preventive, and promotive mental health activities to a more affordable health and community workforce provides a sustainable solution to address this barrier (Patel, 2009; Patel, Chowdhary, Rahman & Verdeli, 2011). Rahman et al. (2000) make the case that services should involve all agencies concerned with child health and well-being for them to be effective. Specialized, primary, and community care services each have a role to play.

Specialized Care

Mental health professionals and specialist workers such as psychiatrists, neurologists, psychiatric nurses, psychologists, mental health social workers, and occupational therapists are rare in many low-income countries, with psychiatrists often numbering less than one per million in the population (Rahman et al., 2000). In Africa (outside of South Africa) there are fewer than ten child and adolescent psychiatrists (WHO, 2005a). Integrating specialized services for mental health into primary health care has the potential to improve access to mental health services and treatment of comorbid physical conditions (WHO & Wonca Working Party on Mental Health, 2008).

Primary Care

Decentralizing models of mental health care will require training primary care providers to provide screening for child and adolescent mental disorders, as well as delivering these services. The professionals that children and adolescents come into contact with are usually doctors, nurses and lay health workers with a limited understanding of children and adolescent mental disorders. Most primary health care facilities in LAMIC do not currently have the skills capacity to provide appropriate interventions for children and adolescents. Providing mental health services through this platform alone will be insufficient. Haines et al. (2007) provide two reasons in support of this argument. First, facility-based services often emphasise only curative care and neglect prevention. Second, children from poor families are less likely or unable to access these health facilities. Unless barriers to both preventive and curative care are addressed and care is brought closer to patients, marginalized at-risk populations will continue to be marginalized (Darmstadt et al., 2005).

Community Care

Increasingly, community-based approaches to care that incorporate good child mental health practices are seen as being feasible in LAMIC (Rahman et al., 2000). Extending the reach of the public health system through a well-trained and supported community health workforce is a crucial step to increasing equity in health care for vulnerable populations (Technical Task Force Report, n.d.). Using community health workers (CHWs) to provide services to address the needs of CAMH has the potential to alleviate the overburdened primary care health system. Numerous platforms are available in communities to reach children and adolescents such as after-school programs, clinics, community centers, orphanages, schools, and residential settings. Community-based systems of care facilitate access to services and allow children and adolescents to be treated in the context of their families, schools, and local communities (WHO, 2005b). Public schools have been identified as a primary site for the delivery of child and adolescent mental health services (WHO, 2005a). The community health workforce can function as the first point in care for communities. CHWs are able to function as the critical link to more clinically skilled workers for more complicated illness or health needs (Technical Task Force Report, n.d.). Investing in new cadres of community health workers should form a major part of strategies to reach the poor who are less likely to use formal health facilities.

Collaboration between service delivery systems and mobilizing a variety of platforms to address CAMH needs is essential for scaling up of promotion, prevention, and intervention strategies, as indicated in table 5.1. Creating a more sustainable mental health workforce requires an effective mix of skills through multidisciplinary collaboration. In the light of current human resource shortage and structural barriers to care one possible solution is the concept of "task shifting."

TASK SHIFTING

The shortage of human resources for mental health impedes the potential scale-up of treatment and provision of care. In Sub-Saharan Africa, thirty-seven of the fifty-seven countries face health worker shortages (WHO, 2006a). The HIV/AIDS epidemic has fueled the health workforce crisis. Sub-Saharan Africa has only 3 percent of the worlds' health workers but the highest prevalence of HIV/AIDS in the world (WHO, 2008). Other factors fueling the human resource shortages include brain drain and the migration of professionals, poor morale, and lack of appropriate incentives (Zachariah et al., 2009). Inequalities are seen between countries but manifest as inequitable health care staff distribution within countries as well, skewing benefits toward both wealthy countries and wealthy urban areas within poor countries (Patel, 2009; Zachariah et al., 2009).

A response to this human resource crisis has been the call for task-shifting in health care services. In 2006, the WHO proposed the Treat, Train, Retain (TTR) strategy to strengthen and expand health workforces in low-income countries which was accompanied by a set of guidelines to provide support for its implementation (WHO, 2006b). While TTR aims to address the human resources crisis for all health issues, it specifically addresses health worker shortages in the context of HIV/AIDS.

Task shifting is defined as the delegation of health care tasks to existing or new cadres with either less training or narrowly tailored training (Zachariah et al., 2009). When task shifting occurs, specific tasks that were previously performed by higher-level cadres are shifted or delegated to lower-level cadres (Zachariah et al., 2009; WHO, 2008). Where appropriate, medical and health service tasks are moved to health workers with shorter training and fewer qualifications. This may occur within the health system, such as when tasks carried out by physicians are taken up by nurses (Lehmann, 2009; Dovlo, 2004). Task shifting also includes the creation of new professional or nonprofessional cadres, with tasks being shifted from workers with more general training to workers who receive specific, competency-based training. At this level, tasks can be delegated outside of the formal health system to trained lay community members, such as CHWs and caregivers (Lehmann, 2009). Through task shifting, non-specialist health workers can be trained to provide health care services under the supervision of specialists. Task shifting serves as a mechanism to compensate for the shortage of specialists in LAMIC, facilitates scaling up of health services at minimal cost and ease bottlenecks in service delivery (WHO 2006b; WHO 2008).

The idea of task shifting is not a novel concept. Informal skill delegation emerged because of unfulfilled needs in rural and remote areas (Dovlo, 2004). In the Congo in the 1950s, nurses were trained to perform surgery (White, Thorpe & Maine, 1987). In his review on task shifting in Africa, Dovlo (2004) describes an illiterate Ethiopian woman trained to repair vesico-vaginal fistulae while working with an Australian missionary doctor. The first CHW programs were China's barefoot doctors and Thailand's village health volunteers and communicators who were involved in primary health care programs and distribution of essential drugs for marginalized communities (Sringeryuang, Hongvivatana & Pradabmuk, 1995). After some 85 percent of its doctors emigrated, Mozambique began to utilize surgical/obstetric technicians (*tecnicos de cirurgýa*) who could independently perform surgery (Vas, Bergstrom, Vaz, Langa & Bugalho, 1999).

Task shifting may increase efficiency and cost-effective service delivery when lower-level cadres are able to produce the same quality as higher-level cadres. Another objective of task shifting is to reduce the time needed to scale up the health workforce, because the cadres performing the shifted tasks require less training. The efficiency gain from changing the skill mix of health workers results in increased patient access, a reduction in health worker training and wage bill costs, and a reduction in the health workforce needs-based shortage (Lehmann, Van Damme, Barten & Sanders, 2009).

Task shifting has been effective in a variety of contexts. In Kenya, no significant clinical differences were found between HIV/AIDS patients who received clinic-based antiretroviral therapy care versus primarily community-based care (Selke et al., 2010). The *tecnicos de cirurgýa* in Mozambique produced similar patient outcomes as compared to physician obstetricians and gynecologists, but their cost of surgery was estimated to be one-quarter of physician specialists (Kruk, Pereira, Vaz, Bergstrom & Galea, 2007). Huicho and colleagues found that the number of years of pre-service training was generally not associated with the appropriate assessment, diagnosis, and treatment of young children in Bangladesh, Brazil, Tanzania, and Uganda (Huicho, Scherpbier, Nkowane & Victora, 2008). These findings demonstrate how task shifting can be implemented as a pragmatic response to health workforce shortages in a variety of settings.

Task shifting is intended to help produce a strengthened and flexible health workforce that can respond to the changing landscape of public health needs. A well-implemented community health workforce can improve health-seeking behaviours and provide low-cost interventions, enabling improvements in the continuum of care (Technical Task Force Report, n.d.). In the following section we discuss how task shifting has the potential to reduce the barriers to care in the field of mental health, with specific reference to CAMH services.

Task Shifting in Mental Health

In their review of the current situation on human resources for mental health care, Kakuma et al. (2011) report that all low-income countries and about two-thirds of middle-income countries had fewer mental health workers available to deliver core mental health interventions. A number of major trails to date have shown that individuals with no mental health background can deliver psychological treatments effectively with relatively little training and continued supervision (Patel et al. 2011; Van Ginneken et al. 2011). Social workers and nurses in primary health care clinics provided a collaborative stepped-care intervention that improved outcomes for depressed women in Chile (Arya et al. 2003). Based on this successful trial, Patel et al. (2010) used the same approach using trained lay health counsellors for treating depressive and anxiety disorders. The intervention improved recovery rates for patients with common mental disorders in public primary care settings. A community-based rehabilitation program using local village health groups was more effective than standard outpatient care for chronic schizophrenia in India (Chatterjee, Patel, Chatterjee &Weis, 2003).

Opportunities for Task Shifting in Child and Adolescent Mental Health

In LAMIC there is a lack of trained individuals to staff even basic child and adolescent mental health treatment facilities and certainly not sufficient to provide services across the continuum of care (WHO, 2005a). Incorporating community-focused mental health care by shifting tasks to non-specialist mental health workers, teachers, or community workers is a valuable strategy to address barriers to both preventative and curative care. The interventions discussed in this section were chosen to provide evidence of how task shifting can be implemented effectively to improve outcomes in CAMH in LAMIC. Universal and selective interventions aimed at maternal, child, and adolescent health are included, justified by the need for a continuum of care.

Prevention strategies can either be directed toward all children in a particular setting (universal) or focus on children who are at increased risk of developing mental health problems (selective/indicated). Population-wide preventative measures can markedly reduce morbidity from mental ill health among children (Eisenburg, 1992). A number of preventative interventions in LAMIC focus on improving maternal health and reducing child mortality and morbidity, with a larger body of evidence available on the effectiveness of these programs. These are important, since improvement in this sphere will be important in determining mental health outcomes for children. Task shifting through low-cost community-based interventions has been shown to be an effective strategy to address common maternal and child health issues (Technical Task Force Report, n.d.). Delivering home visits to improve maternal, newborn, and child health was originally a task developed for nurses. Due to a shortage of trained nurses in LAMIC, these tasks have further been shifted to the cadre of CHWs and this strategy has proven to be effective (Rotherham-Borus et al., 2011).

The Technical Task Force Report (n.d.) lists a variety of interventions that can be provided through CHWs such as promoting immunisation uptake, exclusive breastfeeding, ARV usage; treating for common ailments such as malaria, diarrhea, and pneumonia; providing home-based neo-natal care and family planning. A Cochrane review found that lay health workers increased uptake of immunizations and breastfeeding, improved TB treatment outcomes, and prevented child morbidity and mortality in comparison to standard care (Lewin et al. 2010). CHWs are now trained to provide not only services targeting physical health of mothers and children but psychosocial interventions as well. Intervention strategies incorporating mental health into existing programs for maternal and child health are now emerging, as was done with Philani's Mentor Moth-

PHILANI PLUS (+): THE MENTOR MOTHER COMMUNITY HEALTH WORKER PROGRAMME

Philani is a NGO operating in 150 township neighborhoods that use CHWs (Mentor Mothers) to make home visits aimed at improving infant and child nutritional status and development. The original Philani Intervention Programme has a thirty-year history of sustainable home-based support for pregnant women and malnourished children (le Roux et al., 2010; le Roux et al., 2011). The Philani Plus (+) Intervention Program was conceived to integrate into the existing Philani Intervention Program to address other challenges such as HIV, alcohol abuse and poor mental health. Mentor Mothers are trained over a two-month period, making home visits on four days and attending supervision one day weekly. Twice monthly, a supervisor attends the home visits with the Mentor Mother. Mobile phones with a study-specific application act as a monitoring and supervision system. Scales and growth charts are used to identify malnourished children; pregnant women are encouraged to attend antenatal sessions and exclusively breastfeed, abstain from alcohol and smoking during pregnancy, and take all medicine prescribed in antenatal care. In a cluster randomized controlled trial, compared to women in the control group, women living with HIV receiving the intervention were more likely to complete tasks to prevent vertical transmission, use one feeding method for six months, avoid birth-related medical complications, and were less likely to have stunted infants. Among all mothers, compared to control mothers, mothers receiving the Philani intervention were more likely to use condoms consistently, breastfed exclusively for six months, and were also less likely to have stunted infants. The children of women who were antenatally depressed in the Philani intervention group were also more often in the normative weight and height for age over time, and have higher IQ at eighteen months compared to women depressed during this period who did not receive the Philani intervention (le Roux et al., 2013). This program demonstrates the potential for CHW home visits to effectively identify, engage, and deliver interventions to mothers where multiple health risks are present at the community level.

ers from South Africa (see case study 1) and the Lady Health Worker Programme in Pakistan (Rahman, Malik, Sikander, Roberts & Creed, 2008).

The Lady Health Worker program offers coverage to more than 80 percent of Pakistan's rural population, providing mainly preventative maternal and child health care and education. An intervention for mothers diagnosed with depression based on CBT-principles was integrated into the routine work of the Lady Health Workers. With brief training and on-going supervision, these CHWs provided the Thinking Healthy Programme to mothers diagnosed with depression. The program more than halved the rate of depression in prenatally depressed women, resulting in less disability and improved overall functioning (Rahman, Malik, Sikander, Roberts & Creed, 2008).

Although evidence of effective mental health interventions aimed specifically at children and adolescents in low-resource settings is limited, there is increasing evidence that prevention strategies focused on early stimulation, mother-child interaction, parenting, and child skills development can benefit the mental health of children both concurrently and in the long term (Kieling et al., 2011).

Psychosocial Interventions Using CHWs: Successful Prevention Studies

Mental health promotion through enhancement of parenting can strengthen protective factors for mental health outcomes in children and adolescents. In a peri-urban community in South Africa, trained women (mothers themselves) from the community provided a fifteen-session mother-infant intervention aimed at improving sensitive responsive interactions (Cooper, Tomlinson, Molteno, Swartz & Murray, 2002). These women received training in basic parenting and counseling skills and received weekly group supervision by an experienced community clinical psychologist. Women receiving the home-based intervention were more sensitive in engagement with their infants, expressing more positive affect than mothers in the control group.

In Ethiopia, health and community workers were trained to provide the More Intelligent and Sensitive Children (MISC) intervention, resulting in improved quality of mother-child interactions and higher frequency of positive affect (Klein & Rye, 2004). Both these factors are associated with long-term positive outcomes for infants. Trained CHWs conducted home-visits to enhance interactions between mothers and their children in Kingston, Jamaica. Stimulation comprised weekly one-hour home visits by CHWs, with the objective of improving mother-child interactions through play. Children receiving stimulation in infancy were less anxious, had fewer symptoms of depression, better self-esteem, and fewer attention problems than their non-stimulated counterparts and less likely to have been suspended from school or expelled than those who had not received stimulation (Walker, Chang, Powell, Simonoff & Grantham-McGregor, 2006).

Task Shifting in Primary Care Services

Universal maternal and child health services can also be used as a platform to deliver interventions aimed at improving child mental health outcomes. In a previously under-served rural area of South Africa, Pillay and Lockhat (1997) engaged local resources by training local primary care nurses and other workers to identify and manage children with uncomplicated psychological problems. The authors, both clinical psychologists, supported the primary care staff through their own clinics and gave consultations to children with mental disorders in communities at a distance of up to two hundred kilometers from their hospital base. Non-specialized health workers have been trained to provide interventions for mothers of children with behavior problems through local health and social service centers in Lebanon. Fayyad and colleagues (2010) in a non-controlled trial adapted eight training sessions for mothers and the training for parents provided effective tools to use with difficult children, resulting in significant improvement in children's behavioral ratings and positive parenting.

Engaging Schools and Teachers to Address CAMH Needs

Schools can be used to bridge the gap between need and utilization for children who would otherwise not have access to mental health services, in providing both universal and selective school-based interventions. Training parents and teachers and implementing school-based psychosocial interventions is an essential task-shifting strategy that can improve child behaviour outcomes. The Jamaica pilot study of the "Incredible Years Teacher Training" program (Baker-Henningham, Walker, Powell & Gardner, 2009a, 2009b) provided professional development for teachers in implementing socio-emotional skills in the curriculum and showed benefits in ratings of children's appropriate classroom behavior, reporting fewer aggressive and disruptive acts (Baker-Henningham, Walker, Powell & Gardner, 2009a, 2009b). Similarly, teachers were trained to implement a school-based program named Zippy's Friends that assisted children in developing coping and social skills. A study of children in Denmark and Lithuania showed that skills of cooperation, self-control, assertion, and empathy all increased in groups receiving the program compared to groups that did not (Mishara & Ystgaard, 2006).

Selective interventions targeting problems (rather than preventively) have also been implemented in the school setting. In China, the school engaged parents in life-skills education to reduce behavior problems in third-grade students (Lin, Wang & Wu, 2007). Life-skills education effectively reduced children's behavior problems both at school and at home, especially with regard to antisocial behavior (Lin, Wang & Wu, 2007). A Chinese RCT using the Penn Optimism program based on CBT principles showed a significant reduction of depressive symptoms in 220 subclinically depressed school children post-treatment and at the three- and six-month follow-up (Yu & Seligman, 2002). Classroom-based interventions can provide relief to children affected by trauma and violence in areas where psychosocial services are otherwise unavailable and uses service providers who form part of child and adolescent natural ecologies.

In conflict-affected Nepal, community interventionists who were trained during a fifteen-day skill-based course and supervised by an experienced counselor provided a classroom-based intervention for children with elevated psychosocial distress (Jordans et al., 2010). The intervention reduced psychosocial difficulties and aggression among boys and increased pro-social behavior among girls but did not result in a reduction of psychiatric symptoms of PTSD, anxiety, and depression (Jordans et al., 2010). Interventions such as these should ideally be implemented in conjunction with more specialized services to treat more severe cases.

Engaging Community Members to Address CAMH Needs

The active involvement and empowerment of communities may have positive effects on mental health outcomes for children and adolescents by providing support to at-risk groups in the community, changing health beliefs, raising awareness, or improving access to health and other services. For example, where resources to develop specialist care for children with learning or developmental disabilities are scarce, a solution may be to facilitate the primary care giver to take on the role of "therapist." In India, parents were trained by psychologists on aspects of child rearing skills and behavioral techniques that improved their knowledge and attitude towards intellectual disability as well as care management skills (Russel, John & Lakshmanan, 1999). In Vietnam, teachers were mobilized to provide a home-visit service to preschool-aged children with intellectual disabilities that was effective in improving personal care skills and motor skills compared to the control group (Shin et al., 2009). In South Africa, trained youth caregivers provided psychosocial support and HIV education to primary school students living in vulnerable settings, facilitating referrals to more comprehensive community services when needed. Students' participation in the program was associated with

A THREE-TIER SCHOOL-BASED PROGRAM FOR WAR-EXPOSED ADOLESCENTS

The Bosnian war claimed 100,000 lives, resulting in multiple trauma exposures and severe hardship for civilians. Surveys of children and adolescents across the region revealed high rates of violent deaths of parents or family members and associated distress reactions. During a needs assessment reviewing the availability of psychosocial services to Bosnian children and adolescents, many youths were found to experience persisting symptoms of PTSD, traumatic grief, and functional impairment due to the major disruptions in their developmental trajectories. A three-tiered school- and community-based mental health program was implemented with Bosnian secondary students exposed to severe trauma, traumatic bereavement, and adversity. The program was implemented by local school and community professionals aiming to reduce mental distress, promote adaptive functioning, and reduce the risk of mental ill health for this group. The first level of intervention (tier 1) consisted of participation in a classroom-based psycho-education and skills intervention. The second level (tier 2) combined this classroom-based intervention with a manual-based seventeen-session trauma- and grief-focused group treatment consisting of trauma and grief component therapy (TGCT). A small number of very distressed students of acute risk of self-harm were referred to community specialist services (tier 3). School counselors were trained with the support from local mental health professionals, acting as supervisors and consultants. Results from a randomized control trial evaluating the intervention indicated that tier 1 was effective in significantly reducing PTSD and depressive symptoms, with tier 2 showing even higher improvements in the aforementioned symptoms as well as improvement in maladaptive grief. PTSD and depressive symptoms continued to improve between post-treatment and four-month follow-up. This multi-tier mental health intervention demonstrates that creating a professional support network between school and community services can be an effective tool in preventing mental ill health for such at-risk groups.

improved HIV-related knowledge, more frequent communication about AIDS, and more accepting attitudes toward people infected and affected by HIV (Nelson et al., 2008). In Rwanda, adult mentors have been used to provide support for orphans and vulnerable children as a way of involving communities in order to address their own needs and minimize adverse outcomes for vulnerable groups.

An experimental community-based drug intervention was implemented in nineteen villages in China that aimed to reduce the high prevalence of drug use among males aged eighteen to twenty-nine years. The

ADULT MENTORSHIP PROGRAMME FOR YOUTH HEADED HOUSEHOLDS IN GIKONGORO PROVINCE

Rwanda has one of the world's highest percentages of orphans among children seventeen years and younger (17 percent), with large numbers of youth-headed households (YYH). The HIV epidemic, combined with the ongoing effects of the genocide, left many children living without adult care or supervision. These young people are "left behind" by not only parents and other caregivers who have died but often also by extended families, communities, and formal structures. One model of community-based psychosocial support is the mentorship model, which utilized trained adult volunteers from the local community as mentors to children and youth living without adult care. Through regular home visits, adult volunteers from the local community are trained and supported to monitor the well-being of these children and youth, provide guidance and transfer life skills, help ensure health and safety, and act as advocates on behalf of the YHH. The project is intended to strengthen the supportive environment and mitigate the impacts of disrupted care-giving structures and marginalization. Mentors received ongoing support and supervision from World Vision Rwanda. High levels of psychosocial distress, especially depressive symptoms, were present at baseline among these youths. The intervention was associated with improvements in psychosocial outcomes. Youths who participated in the mentorship program showed a significant decrease in feelings of marginalization and depressive symptoms compared to youth participants who did not receive the intervention. This programme indicates that through training and ongoing support and supervision, community members were able to effectively address a mental health-related need in their community by providing front-line care and support to children and youth affected by AIDS.

prevention program actively involved local community members in the intervention activities; village leaders and village health workers were trained. Not only were they responsible for implementing the intervention but they played a key role in the development of the intervention strategies. Intervention efforts (including drug prevention messages, school programs, visits to detoxifications centers) were successful in reducing the incidence of new drug users and improving knowledge and attitudes compared to the villages in the control group (Wu, Detels, Zhang, Li & Li, 2002). This indicates the value of such an approach for preventing children and adolescents from developing problematic behavior later in life.

These interventions provide examples of innovative and effective strategies to expand mental health services for mothers, children, and adolescents to primary care settings and into the community. Task shifting is essential to increase capacity and health care coverage where health systems face systematic underfunding and lack of qualified staff. Furthermore, it enables the provision of a continuum of care in its potential to bridge mental health issues with existing public health priorities and address the physical and environmental difficulties to improve mental health outcomes of children and adolescents (WHO, 2005b). A perspective emphasising continuum of care through a combination of platforms is likely to be a more acceptable vehicle for intervention than a focus on any single condition or disease entity. Comprehensive strategies that begin early in life and continue over time are urgently needed.

A number of factors need to be considered for task shifting to be successful and sustainable. When tasks have been shifted from traditional professional cadres (e.g., specialists, doctors or nurses) to new professional cadres, most studies compare the new cadre's productivity and patient outcomes to the traditional cadre's. However, Fulton et al. (2010) point out that the appropriate comparison is between the results from the care received by the new cadre and the results from the care the patient would have received—if any care at all—had the new cadre not been available. Before programs are scaled-up, more robust evidence is needed regarding the effectiveness and sustainability of such interventions through alternative health workers. Many of the findings presented here were based on RCTs, which Lewin (2006) argues have higher levels of organization and support than those usually available outside of research settings. Supportive management, appropriate supervision and availability of infrastructural support are therefore critical issues for program success (Haines et al., 2007).

Training is a vital component of any task-shifting initiative. Kakuma et al. (2011) reported that overall short-term training by specialist mental health professionals with ongoing supervision can improve confidence, detection, treatment, and treatment adherence of individuals with mental disorders and reduce caregiver burden. While task shifting offers the potential for significant gains in mental health outcomes of children and adolescents, scaling up of these interventions will require continued linkages to existing service delivery systems. Tasks need to be *shared* and not "dumped" onto lower level workers, since CHWs cannot provide comprehensive care for all community needs. Funds need to be allocated for both recruitment and training of the task-sharing workforce, while providing infrastructure to enable them to fulfill tasks.

Task shifting is in line with growing evidence that alternative health worker cadres can deliver aspects of mental health care at primary and community levels where specialized personnel are limited. While task shifting holds significant promise for improving population level mental health across LAMIC, it should not be seen as a panacea for the human resources challenge faced by LAMIC (Philips, Zachariah & Venis, 2008). Task shifting alone will not put an end to the shortage of health workers, but it may offer the only realistic possibility of expanding health workforce capacity fast enough to meet the need for scaling up of services (WHO, 2008a). The studies described here demonstrate that it is possible to design and implement interventions that are efficacious and relatively low-cost. What is needed is rigorous evidence of the utilization of task shifting within CAMH services, and evidence of this at scale.

REFERENCES

Araya, R., Rojas, G., Fritsch, R., Gaete, J., Rojas, M., Simon, G. & Peters, T. J. (2003). Treating depression in primary care in low-income women in Santiago, Chile: A randomised controlled trial. *Lancet* 361, 995–1000.

Baker-Henningham, H., Walker, S. P., Powell, C. & Gardner, J. M. (2009a). A pilot study of the Incredible Years Teacher Training program and a curriculum unit on social and emotional skills in community pre-schools in Jamaica. *Child: Care, Health and Development* 35, 624–31.

Baker-Henningham, H., Walker, S. P., Powell, C. & Gardner, J. M. (2009b). Preventing behaviour problems through a universal intervention in Jamaican basic schools: A pilot study. *West Indian Medical Journal* 58, 460–64.

Bang, A. T., Reddy, H. M., Deshmukh, M. D., Baitule, S. B. & Bang, R. A. (2005). Neonatal and infant mortality in the ten years (1993 to 2003) of the Gadchiroli field trial: Effect of home-based neonatal care. *Journal of Perinatology* 25, S92–S107.

Burns, B. J., Costello, E. J., Angold, A., Tweed, D., Stangl, D., Farmer, E. M. & Erklani, A. (1995). Children's mental health services use across services sectors. *Health Affairs* 14, 147–59.

Chatterjee, S., Patel, V., Chatterjee, A. & Weiss, H. A. (2003). Evaluation of a community based rehabilitation model for chronic schizophrenia in rural India. *British Journal of Psychiatry* 182, 57–62. doi: 10.1192/bjp.182.1.57.

Collins, P. Y., Patel, V., Joestl, S. S., March, D., Insel, T. R. & Daar, A. S. (2011). Grand challenges in global mental health. *Nature* 472, 27–30.

Cooper, P., Landman, M., Tomlinson, M., Molteno, C., Swartz, L. & Murray, L. (2002). The impact of a mother-infant intervention in an indigent peri-urban South African context: Pilot study. *British Journal of Psychiatry* 180, 76–81.

Darmstadt, G. L., Bhutta, Z. A., Cousens, S., Adam, T., Walker, N. & de-Bernis, L. (2005). Evidence-based, cost effective interventions: How many newborn babies can we save? *Lancet* 365, 977–88.

Dovlo, D. (2004). Using mid-level cadres as substitutes for internationally mobile health professionals in Africa: A desk review. *Human Resources for Health* 2, 7. doi: 10.1186/1478-4491-2-7.

Eisenberg, L. (1992). Child mental health in the Americas: A public health approach. *Bulletin of PAHO* 26, 230–41.

Eisenberg, L. & Belfer, M. (2009). Prerequisites for global child and adolescent mental health. *Journal of Child Psychology and Psychiatry* 50, 26–35.

Fayyad, J. A., Farah, L., Cassir, Y., Salamoun, M. M. & Karam, E. G. (2010). Dissemination of an evidence-based intervention to parents of children with behavioural problems in a developing country. *European Child and Adolescent Psychiatry* 19, 629–36. doi: 10.1007/s00787-010- 0099-3.

Fulton, B. D., Scheffer, R. M., Sparkes, S. P., Yoonkyung Auh, E., Vujicic, M. & Soucat, A. (2011). Health workforce skill mix and task shifting in low income countries: A review of recent evidence. *Human Resources for Health* 9, 1.

Grantham-McGregor, S., Cheung, Y. B., Cueto, S., Glewwe, P., Richter, L. & Strupp, B: International Child Development Steering Group. (2007). Developmental potential in the first 5 years for children in developing countries. *Lancet* 369, 60–70.

Haines, A., Sanders, D., Lehman, U., Rowe, A., Lawn, J. E., Jan, S., Bhutta, Z. (2007). Achieving child survival goals: Potential contribution of community health workers. *Lancet* 369, 2121-31. doi: 10.1016/S0140-6736(07)60325-0.

Horizons. (2007). *Assessing the psychosocial benefits of a community-based mentoring program for youth-headed households in Rwanda.* Washington, DC: Population Council, World Vision Rwanda, Rwanda School of Public Health, Tulane University School of Public Health and Tropical Medicine.

Huicho. L., Scherpbier, R. W., Nkowane, A. M. & Victora, C. G. (2008). The multicountry evaluation of IMCI Study Group: How much does quality of child care vary between health workers with differing durations of training? An observational multicountry study. *Lancet* 372, 910–16.

Jordans, M. J., Komproe, I. H., Tol, W. A., Kohrt, B. A., Luitel, N. P., Macy, R. D. & de Jong, J. T. (2010). Evaluation of a classroom-based psychosocial intervention in conflict affected Nepal: A cluster randomized controlled trial. *Journal of Child Psychology and Psychiatry* 51, 818–826. doi:10.1111/j.1469-7610.2010.02209.x

Kakuma, R., Minas, H., van Ginneken, N., Dal Poz, M. R., Desiraju, K., Morris, J. E., Scheffler, R. M. (2011). Human resources for mental health care: Current situation and strategies for action. *Lancet* 378, 1654–63. doi: 10.1016/S0140 6736(11)61093-3.

Kessler R. C., Angermeyer, M., Anthony, J. C., de Graaf, R., Demyttenaere, K., Gasquet, I., Bedirhan Üstün, T. (2007). Lifetime prevalence and age-of-onset distributions of mental disorders in the World Health Organization's World Mental Health Survey Initiative. *World Psychiatry* 6, 168–76.

Kieling, C., Baker-Henningham, H., Belfer, M., Conti, G., Ertem, I., Omigbodun, O., Rahman, A. (2011). Child and adolescent mental health worldwide: evidence for action. *Lancet* 378, 1515–25. doi: 10.1016/S0140-6736(11)60745-9.

Klasen, H. & Crombag, A-C. (2013). What works where? A systematic review of child and adolescent mental health interventions for low and middle income countries. *Social Psychiatry and Psychiatric Epidemiology* 48, 595–611. doi: 10.1007/s00127-012 0566-x.

Klein, P. S. & Rye, H. (2004). Interaction-oriented early intervention in Ethiopia: The MISC approach. *Infants and Young Children* 17, 340–54.

Kohn, R., Saxema, S., Levav, I. & Saraceno, B. (2004). The treatment gap in mental health care. *Bulletin of the World Health Organisation* 82, 858–66. doi.org/10.1590/S0042 96862004001100011.

Kruk, M., Pereira, C., Vaz, F., Bergstrom, S. & Galea, S. (2007). Economic evaluation of surgically trained assistant medical officers in performing major obstetric surgery in Mozambique. *British Journal of Obstetrics and Gynaecology* 114, 1253–60.

Layne, C. M., Saltzman, W. R., Poppleton, L., Burlingame, G. M., Pašalić, A., Duraković, E., Pynoos, R. S. (2008). Effectiveness of a school-based group psychotherapy program for war-exposed adolescents: A randomized controlled trial. *Journal of American Academic Child and Adolescent Psychiatry* 47, 1048–62.

Lehmann, U. (2009). Strengthening human resources for primary health care. In P. Barron (Ed.), *South African Health Review 2008* (pp. 163–73). Durban: Health Systems Trust.

Lehmann, U., Van Damme, W., Barten, F. & Sanders, D. (2009). Task shifting: The answer to the human resources crisis in Africa? *Human Resources for Health* 7, 49.

le Roux, I., le Roux, K., Comulada, W. S., Greco, E., Desmond, K., Mbewu, N. & Rotheram Borus, M-J. (2010). Home visits by neighbourhood Mentor Mothers provide timely recovery from childhood malnutrition in South Africa: Results from a randomized controlled trial. *Nutrition Journal* 9, 56.

le Roux, I., le Roux, K., Mbeutu, K., Comulada, W. S., Desmond, K. A. & Rotheram-Borus, M-J. (2011). A randomized controlled trial of home visits by neighbourhood Mentor Mothers to improve children's nutrition in South Africa. *Vulnerable Children and Youth Studies* 6, 91–102.

le Roux, I. M., Tomlinson, M., et al. (2013). Outcomes of home visits for pregnant mothers and their infants: A cluster randomized controlled trial. *AIDS* 27(9): 1461–71.

Lewin, S. A., Babigumira, S. M., Bosch-Capblanch, X., Aja, G., van Wyk, B., Glenton, C., Scheel, I., Zwarenstein, M. & Daniels K. (2006). Lay health workers in primary and community health care: A systematic review of trials.

Lewin, S. A., Munabi-Babigumira, S., Glendon, C., Daniels, K., Bosch-Capblanch, X., van Wyk, B. E., Scheel, I. B. (2010). Lay health workers in primary and community health care for maternal and child health and the management of infectious diseases. *Cochrane Database of Systematic Reviews* 3, CD004015. doi: 10.1002/14651858.CD004015.pub3.

Manandhar, D. S., Osrin, D., Shrestha, B. P., Mesko, N., Morrison, J., Tumbahangphe, K. M., Costello, A. M. (2004). Effect of a participatory intervention with women's groups on birth outcomes in Nepal: Cluster-randomised controlled trial. *Lancet* 364, 970–79.

Mishara, B. & Ystgaard, M. (2006). Effectiveness of a mental health promotion program to improve coping skills in young children: Zippy's friends. *Early Childhood Research Quarterly* 21, 110–23.

Nelson, T. C., Esu-Williams, E., Mchunu, L., Nyamakazi, P., Mnguni, S., Schenk, K., et al. (2008). *Training youth caregivers to provide HIV education and support to orphans and vulnerable children in South Africa.* Horizons Research Summary. Washington: Population Council.

Oveisi, S., Ardabili, H. E., Dadds, M. R., et al. (2010). Primary prevention of parent-child conflict and abuse in Iranian mothers: A randomized-controlled trial. *Child Abuse and Neglect* 34, 206–213.

Patel, V. (2009). The future of psychiatry in low- and middle-income countries. *Psychological Medicine* 39, 1759–62.

Patel, V., Araya, R., Chatterjee, S., Chisholm, D., Cohen, A., de Silva, M., Hosman, C., van Ommeren, M. (2007). Treatment and prevention of mental disorders in low income and middle-income countries. *Lancet* 370, 991–1005.

Patel, V., Boyce, N., Collins, P. Y., Saxena, S. & Horton, R. (2011a). A renewed agenda for global mental health. *Lancet* 378, 1441–42.

Patel, V., Chowdhary, N., Rahman, A. & Verdeli, H. (2011b). Improving access to psychological treatments: Lessons from developing countries. *Behaviour Research and Therapy* 49, 523–28.

Patel, V., Flisher, A. J., Nikapota, A. & Malhotra, S. (2008). Promoting child and adolescent mental health in low and middle income countries. *Journal of Child Psychology and Psychiatry* 49, 313–334. doi: 10.1111/j.1469-7610.2007.01824.x.

Patel, V., Weiss, H. A., Chowdhary, N., Naik, S., Pednekar, S., Chatterjee, S., Kirkwood, B. R. (2010). Effectiveness of an intervention led by lay health counsellors for depressive and anxiety disorders in primary care in Goa, India (MANAS): A cluster randomised controlled trial. *Lancet* 376, 2086–2095. doi: 10.1016/S0140 6736(10)61508-5.

Philips, M., Zachariah, R. & Venis, S. (2008). Task shifting for antiretroviral treatment delivery in sub-Saharan Africa: Not a panacea. *Lancet* 371, 682–84.

Pillay, A. L. & Lockhat, M. R. (1997). Developing community mental health services for children in South Africa. *Social Science and Medicine* 45, 1493–1501.

Rahman, A., Malik, A., Sikander, S., Roberts, C. & Creed, F. (2008). Cognitive behaviour therapy-based intervention by community health workers for mothers with depression and their infants in rural Pakistan: A cluster-randomised controlled trial. *Lancet* 372, 902–9.

Rahman, A., Mubbashar, M., Harrington, R. & Gater, R. (2000). Annotation: Developing child mental health services in developing countries. *Journal of Child Psychology and Psychiatry* 41, 539–46.

Rotheram-Borus, M., le Roux, I. M., Tomlinson, M., Mbewu, N., Comulada, W. S., le Roux, K., Swendeman, D. (2011). Philani Plus (+): A Mentor Mothers community health worker home visiting program to improve maternal and infants' outcomes. *Prevention Science* 12, 372–88. doi: 10.1007/s11121-011-0238-1.

Russell, P. S., al John, J. K. & Lakshmanan, J. L. (1999). Family intervention for intellectually disabled children: Randomised controlled trial. *British Journal of Psychiatry* 174, 254–58. doi:10.1192/bjp. 174.3.254 [57].

Sanders, D. (2010). The missing link: Saving children's lives through family and community care. World Vision International Policy Briefing, World Vision International.

Selke, H. M., Kimaiyo, S., Sidle, J. E., Vedanthan, R., Tierney, W. M., Shen, C., Wools Kaloustian, K. (2010). Task-Shifting of antiretroviral delivery from health care workers to persons living with HIV/AIDS: Clinical outcomes of a community-based program in Kenya. *Journal of Acquired Immune Deficiency Syndromes* 55, 483–90.

Shin, J. Y., Nhan, N. V., Lee, S. B., Crittenden, K. S., Flory, M. & Hong, H. T. D (2009). The effects of a home-based intervention for young children with intellectual disabilities in Vietnam. *Journal of Intellectual Disability Research* 53, 339–52. doi:10.1111/j.1365-2788. 2008.01151.x.

Sringernyuang, L., Hongvivatana, T. & Pradabmuk, P. (1995). Implications of community health workers distributing drugs: A case study of Thailand. Geneva: World Health Organisation.

Sweet, M. A. & Appelbaum, M. I. (2004). Is home visiting an effective strategy? A meta- analytic review of home visiting programs for families with young children. *Child Development* 75, 1435–56. doi:10.1111/j.1467-8624.2004.00750.x.

Technical Task Force Report (n.d). Technical Task Force Report: One Million Community Health Workers. *The Earth Institute, Columbia University.* Retrieved August 27, 2013, from http://www.millenniumvillages.org/uploads/ReportPaper/1mCHW_TechnicalTaskF orceReport.pdf.

Thurman, T. R., Snider, L., Boris, N., Kalisa, E., Mugarira, E. N., Ntaganira, J. & Browne, L. (2006). Psychosocial support and marginalization of youth-headed households in Rwanda. *AIDS Care* 18, 220–29. doi: 10.1080/09540120500456656.

Tomlinson, M. (2010). Family-centred HIV intervention: Lessons from the field of parental depression. *Journal of the International AIDS Society* 13, S9–S17.

Tomlinson, M., Doherty, T., Jackson, D., Lawn, J. E., Ijumba, P., Colvin, M., Chopra, M. (2011). An effectiveness study of an integrated, community-based package for maternal, newborn, child and HIV care in South Africa: Study protocol for a randomised control trial. *Trials* 12, 236.

Van Ginneken, N., Tharyan, P., Lewin, S., Rao, G. N., Romeo, R. & Patel, V. (2011). Non specialist health worker interventions for mental health care in low- and middle income countries (Protocol). *Cochrane Database of Systematic Reviews* 11. doi: 10.1002/14651858.CD009149.

Vaz, F., Bergstrom, S., Vaz, M., Langa, J. & Bugalho, A. (1999). Training medical assistants for surgery: Policy and practice. *Bulletin of the World Health Organization* 77, 688–91.

Walker, S. P., Chang, S. M., Powell, C. A., Simonoff, E. & Grantham-McGregor, S. M. (2006). Effects of psychosocial stimulation and dietary supplementation in early childhood on psychosocial functioning in late adolescence: Follow-up of randomised controlled trial. *British Medical Journal* 333, 472.

Wang, Y., Liu, C. & Wang, Y. F. (2007). Effectiveness of social skills training among children with behaviour problems: A randomized controlled trial. *Beijing Da Xue Xue Bao* 39, 315–58 (in Chinese).

White, S. M., Thorpe, R. G. & Maine, D. (1987). Emergency obstetric surgery performed by nurses in Zaire. *Lancet* 2, 612–13.
World Health Organization (2003). Caring for children and adolescents with mental disorders: Setting WHO directions. Geneva: WHO Press.
World Health Organization. (2005a). Child and adolescent Atlas: Resources for child and adolescent mental health. Geneva: World Health Organization.
World Health Organization. (2005b). Child and adolescent mental health policies and plans: Mental Health Policy and Service Guidance Package. Geneva: World Health Organization.
World Health Organization. (2006a). The World Health Report 2006—Working together for health. Geneva: World Health Organization.
World Health Organisation. (2006b). Treat, train, retrain: The AIDS and health workforce plan. Geneva: World Health Organization.
World Health Organization. (2008). Task shifting: Rational distribution of tasks among health workforce teams: global recommendations and guidelines. Geneva: World Health Organization.
WHO & Wonca Working Party on Mental Health (2008). What is primary care mental health? Wonca/WHO Primary Care Mental Health Factsheet. *Health in Family Medicine* 5, 9–13.
Wu, Z., Detels, R., Zhang, J., Li, V. & Li, J. (2002). Community-based trial to prevent drug use among youths in Yunnan, China. *American Journal of Public Health* 92, 1952–57.
Yu, D. & Seligman, M. (2002). Preventing depressive symptoms in Chinese children. *Prevention Treatment* 5, 1–39.
Zachariah, R., Ford, N., Philips, M., Lynch, S., Massaquoi, M., Janssens, V. & Harries, A. D. (2009). Task shifting in HIV/AIDS: Opportunities, challenges and proposed actions for sub-Saharan Africa. *Transactions of the Royal Society for Tropical Medicine and Hygiene* 103, 549–58.

6

What Works Where?

A Systematic Review of Child and Adolescent Mental Health Interventions for Low- and Middle-Income Countries

Henrikje Klasen, Anne-Claire Crombag, and Koen Stolk

INTRODUCTION

Child and adolescent mental health (CAMH) problems are common, frequently associated with high levels of distress and impairment, and often treatable. Globally about 10–20 percent of children and adolescents suffer from a disabling mental illness. Suicide is the third leading cause of death among adolescents in India and China, and for young people neuropsychiatric disorders are a leading cause of health-related burden accounting for 15–30 percent of their lost disability adjusted life years (DALYs) (Lopez et al., 2006; Kieling et al., 2011). Common childhood psychiatric problems such as behavioral disorders, ADHD, anxiety, and depression have been linked to school failure, criminality, alcohol and substance misuse, accidents, self-harm, (sexual) risk-taking behavior, and unwanted pregnancies. These problems do not end as children grow up but often result in serious social and occupational dysfunction in adult life. In addition, about 50 percent of adult mental health problems begin in youngsters, and reducing the duration of untreated psychiatric disorders by directing more resources to youngsters could improve adult outcome significantly (Patel, 2007a). There is emerging evidence from health economics in low- and middle-income countries (LAMIC) (Miller et al., 2013) that investment in mental health at the beginning of a person's life might yield enormous returns throughout the child's life and into adulthood. Furthermore, the impact and (economic) burden of CAMH problems is not restricted to the affected child but extends to carers, siblings, families, schools, and whole communities in the present as well as the future.

However, resources are scarce in LAMIC and the gap between need and actual provision in CAMH is even higher than in general adult mental health services. The size of the evidence base is illustrative of this gap. Of all mental health treatment trials carried out worldwide by 2007 only a tenth (1,521 studies) were carried out in LAMICs. For children the situation is much worse as only about 1 percent of psychiatric trials carried out in LAMIC specifically addressed CAMH problems (Patel et al., 2007a). Reasons for this neglect and possible ways to address this have been widely discussed, but research and service development remains hampered by lack of government policy, inadequate funding, and a dearth of trained clinicians (Kieling et al., 2011; Patel, 2007b).

Much CAMH research in high-income countries (HIC) countries in the past decades has focused on developing and evaluating interventions, and there is now robust evidence for effective treatments for many child psychiatric problems. For more chronic disorders, such as autism and cognitive disabilities, there are still no cures but better understanding of the disorders has led to improvements in care and management, leading to more independence and social inclusion of affected children and better educational, behavioral, and emotional outcomes. The argument for addressing CAMH problems is not only economic but also ethical and humanitarian with a responsibility to protect and care for this vulnerable group and allow them the best chances of reaching their potential (Collins et al., 2011). While there is general consensus that more research is needed, service provision cannot, and in reality does not, wait for this evidence to become available. Many LAMICs are beginning to implement child mental health policies, and humanitarian agencies increasingly carry out psychosocial care programs for children.

The challenge at this point is to make best use of the available evidence and use scarce resources in the most (cost-) effective way. Currently, all too often this does not happen. Disproportionate amounts of funding go into hospitals or centers serving very few individuals or into private care for those who can afford it. Directly applying interventions developed in HIC might work if the evidence is very robust (multiple RCTs, i.e., randomized controlled trials, in various cultural settings and meta-analyses) especially in the case of more biological disorders. However, cultural differences in the expression and experience of illness, as well as socioeconomic factors and differences in health systems limit the generalizability of many HIC findings. Furthermore, many of the interventions developed in HIC require a large input of highly trained staff, thus making them unfeasible for LAMIC. More importantly there is a growing body of increasingly well-designed intervention studies, including some RCTs emerging from LAMIC (Lund et al., 2011).

The aim of this chapter is to identify the most promising interventions and the most urgent research gaps in the area of global CAMH interventions. This is done by carrying out a systematic review of the evidence from RCTs in LAMIC on treatment and prevention of CAMH problems including childhood developmental disorders. RCTs are generally regarded as the best test of the efficacy of preventive or therapeutic interventions. They require rigorously controlled circumstances which in real-life settings, particularly in LAMIC, are difficult to achieve. Although we are aware of the challenges and limitations in carrying out RCTs of CAMH interventions in LAMIC, we chose this focus as an initial step to gain an overview of the field. The diversity of problems treated and interventions used does not yet allow for quantitative analysis of this evidence.

Where data from child and adolescent RCTs in LAMIC were not available we have also drawn selectively on level 1a evidence, i.e., systematic reviews (CEBM 2009) from HIC, program evaluations from LAMIC (e.g., community-based rehabilitation—CBR), and lessons learned from adult RCTs in LAMIC (e.g., for treating anxiety and depression).

METHODS

We systematically searched for RCTs and cluster RCTs carried out with children and adolescents in LAMIC searching Embase, PsychInfo, Medline, Pub Med, and the Cochrane database of trials up to April 2013, limiting results to English language, children and adolescent, and controlled studies. In this manner we identified 9,274 trials. We further limited our search to studies including populations from LAMIC as defined by the World Bank (The World Bank Group, 2011) or from poverty areas, yielding 514 studies. We screened the abstracts of these papers and again excluded any that were not directly mental health related, were not RCTs, did not include populations from LAMIC, or did not include children and adolescents. We enhanced our search strategy by checking the identified papers for any cited material we had previously missed and by keyword instead of MeSH term searching. In total we identified sixty-four trials of child and adolescent mental health RCTs and cluster RCTs in LAMIC.

(Further details on all studies, keywords and MeSH terms used are available from the authors.)

RESULTS

Behavioral Disorders

Introduction

"Behavioral disorders" is used by the WHO's mental health gap action program (mhGAP) as an umbrella term including more specific disorders such as oppositional defiant disorder (ODD), conduct disorder (CD), and attention deficit hyperactivity disorder (ADHD). Affected children are characterized by defiant, antisocial, or aggressive behaviors, sometimes resulting in CD who in turn are characterised by more serious problems such as cruelty, fighting, stealing, lying, running away, and general destructiveness. There may also be varying levels of inattention, impulsivity, and hyperactivity (ADHD). The worldwide prevalence of ADHD among youngsters age eighteen and younger is estimated to be 5.29 percent (Polanczyk et al., 2007). Childhood CD and ADHD significantly increase the risk for low academic achievement, poor employment prospects, and offending.

Evidence from LAMIC

As the term chosen by the WHO is quite broad there is great variation in the studies reported here: some are preventive; others treat manifest problems; some focus on training parents; others are school-based addressing children and/or teachers; and others test pharmacotherapies. Problems treated include general behavior problems, ODD, and ADHD (see table 6.1).

The *parent interventions* varied in intensity and severity of problems treated ranging from two sessions of parent management skills training (Jordans et al., 2012; Oveisi et al., 2010) to comprehensive systemic treatments by U.S. accredited therapists for children with manifest ADHD and behavior problems (Matos, 2009). Most studies found improvements in child behavior, parent-child interaction, and often in parental well-being and frequency of harsh physical punishment of children. Interestingly, some of the programs were much lower in intensity than those usually delivered in HIC but still showed relatively large effects even in the group above nine years of age where comparable programs in HIC work less well (Jordans et al., 2012; Oveisi et al., 2010).

There is also great variation in *school-based programs*. Sometimes unmodified treatment packages from HIC are used with great success but at rather large cost (Baker-Henningham et al., 2009), and sometimes creative mixed methods are developed as in a Brazilian study where school dropout and absenteeism was reduced with an effect size of 0.64 (Graeff-Martins, 2006). Some programs work better in LAMIC than in HIC, such as a thirteen-session universal prevention program for behavioral problems in China working directly with children in school which achieved decreased behavior problems at home post-treatment and at six-month follow-up (Hong, 2011). In contrast, child-focused programs in HIC have shown little effect.

ADHD studies focussed on pharmacotherapy with small RCTs carried out in Brazil and Russia of the short-term effects of methylphenidate (MPH) and atomoxetine showed the intervention group had significantly better improvement than controls (Martenyi et al., 2011; Szobot et al., 2004). As stimulants are often not available, and sometimes banned in LAMIC, it is useful to note that an evaluation of two second-line drugs, clonidine and carbamazepine, found clonidine but not carbamazepine reduced symptoms of hyperactivity and impulsivity but not inattention (Nair, 2009).

Most Robust Evidence from HIC

For young children (nine years or under) parenting approaches are well-established interventions supported by several RCTs, replications and meta-analyses (Taylor, 2008; Santosh, 2008). Several manualized treatment packages, both for individuals and groups of parents, are effective but often require extensive training and supervision to avoid program drift. Parenting programs also improve depression, anxiety/stress, self-esteem, and relationship with spouse/marital adjustment in participating mothers (Barlow, 2004). Sometimes teacher training as well as child social skills groups complement parent training. Effect sizes are moderate to large (0.5-0.8) with enduring effects at up to six-years post-treatment (Collett, 2009). In older children more resource intense multi-modal interventions are often needed, and a Cochrane review showed that parenting and family interventions help reduce arrests and time spent in institutions (Woolfenden, 2001).

For ADHD numerous well-conducted trials have demonstrated that stimulants are an effective treatment for the core symptoms of ADHD as well as benefiting some secondary symptoms such as academic underperformance and difficulties in peer and family interactions (Taylor, 2008; Santosh, 2008). There is also level 1a evidence for the non-stimulant atomoxetine and for tricyclic antidepressants, although they have an inferior risk/benefit ratio. Behavioral parent training, behavioral classroom management, and intensive peer-focused behavioral interventions (e.g., summer camps) are also well-established treatments (Pelham Jr., 2008), while there is less evidence for individual child-focused approaches.

Table 6.1. Randomized controlled trials (RCTs) for behavioral disorders

Setting	*Study design*	*Sample*	*Intervention*	*Comparison group*	*Main results*
Elementary school in China (Hong, 2011)	RCT	417 children out of six classrooms	school-based prevention curriculum of 13-sessions	no intervention	Behavioral problems were significantly lower in the intervention group post-test—and at six-month follow-up.
Primary care clinic in Iran (Oveisi, 2010)	RCT	224 mothers of young children who visit health centers	preventative parenting program of two times two hours based on "SOS! Help for Parents"	no intervention	Significant improvements on measures of parenting (p= .001) and parent-child conflict (p= .001). Improvement maintained at eight-week follow up.
Five pre-schools in Kingston, Jamaica (Baker-Henningham, 2009 (a))	RCT	135 children with behavior problems out of seventeen classrooms	school-based workshops based on "Incredible Years" Teacher Training	no intervention	The effect sizes for the intervention were 0.26 for conduct problems, 0.36 for hyperactivity, and 0.71 for peer problems.
Five pre-schools in Kingston, Jamaica (Baker-Henningham, 2009 (b))	Pilot RCT	135 children with behavior problems out of seventeen classrooms	school-based workshops based on "Incredible Years" Teacher Training	no intervention	Teachers reported increased positive behavior, reduced negative behavior, and increases in the promotion of children's social and emotional skills; children improved appropriate behavior, interest, and enthusiasm.
Kingston, Jamaica (Baker-Henningham, 2012)	RCT	225 children, aged three to six	school-based workshops based on "Incredible Years" Teaching Training	no intervention	Intervention resulted in significantly reduced conduct problems (ES=.42) and increased friendship skills (ES=.74).

Russia (Martenyi, 2010)	RCT	Seventy-two patients aged six to sixteen years with ADHD Meaning unclear as seventy-two had atomoxetine	pharmacotherapy with atomoxetine during six weeks	placebo	Atomoxetine group (n = 72) showed significantly greater improvement than controls (p = .013).
Hospital in South India (Nair, 2009)	RCT	Fifty children with ADHD aged four to twelve years	pharmacotherapy with second-line drug Clonidine	Carbamazepine	Clonidine more effective in improving the hyperactivity (p< .0001) and impulsivity (p= .0006) than carbamazepine. Clonidine can be a safer and cheaper alternative in treatment of children with ADHD.
Taiwan (Gau, 2007)	RCT	106 patients aged six to sixteen years with ADHD	pharmacotherapy with atomoxetine during six weeks	placebo	Significantly greater reductions in ADHD symptoms with atomoxetine according to investigators, parents, and teachers (effect size 0.70). Adverse events were also significantly increased with decreased appetite (36.1%) and nausea (16.6%).

Implications for Practice in LAMIC

There is now evidence that simplified parent training programs, which can be delivered by trained non-specialists, have been successfully modified to work in LAMIC settings. Follow-up periods have been quite short, and maintaining program fidelity can be a big problem. Another difficulty remains the frequent lack of diagnostic capacity in LAMIC. As disruptive behaviors may be related to many other disorders such as ADHD, autistic spectrum disorders, trauma, emotional problems, and learning difficulties, sometimes other approaches may be needed.

For treating ADHD it is likely that the benefits of stimulant medication generalize to LAMIC; however, these medications are not available in many countries, and an inclusion on the WHO list of essential medications should be considered. General recommendations are that stimulant medication should only be prescribed by suitably trained professionals. In their absence psycho-education and parent training groups can be administered by community staff and are likely to bring some improvement.

Trauma

Introduction

Severe traumatic experiences through war, migration, natural disasters, chronic poverty, or loss of a close relative are much more common in LAMIC than in HIC. The risk of developing symptoms of post-traumatic stress disorder (PTSD), chronic symptoms of anxiety, or depression are significantly increased in war-exposed children, with incidences of up to 30–60 percent (Yule, 2008). Idioms of distress, i.e., the way trauma-related symptoms are expressed, may vary cross-culturally (Hinton et al., 2005), and care is needed when using trauma symptom measures cross-culturally. Furthermore, universal prevention or debriefing of all affected individuals immediately after a traumatic event may do more harm than good (Yule, 2008). This was taken into account in the recently developed WHO Guide for Fieldworkers in delivering Psychological First Aid (WHO, 2011). In this section we include studies dealing with children exposed to traumatic events who developed a variety of psychiatric problems including PTSD, anxiety, depression and/or behavioral problems.

Evidence from LAMIC

We found a total of fourteen RCTs focusing on post-traumatic symptomatology benefitting children in LAMIC (see table 6.2).

Almost all published RCTs found some reduction in symptomatology which was usually maintained at three-months follow-up, although their treatment approaches differed quite considerably. Some harnessed culture-specific coping mechanisms and focused strongly on mind-body skills (Gordon et al., 2008; Lesmana et al., 2009); others adapted techniques such as cognitive behavior therapy (CBT) (Tol et al., 2008; Berger, 2009), interpersonal therapy (IPT) (Schaal, 2009; Bolton et al., 2007), narrative exposure therapy (NET) (Ertl et al., 2011; Schaal, 2009; Catani et al., 2009), or writing for recovery (Kalantari et al., 2012) to be delivered by lay counselors in group, classroom, or individual settings. Others worked with mothers to affect both their own and their young children's psychological functioning (Dybdahl, 2001), while others (Tol et al., 2010; Jordans et al., 2010) used an eclectic mix of techniques.

Classroom-Based Intervention (CBI) delivered by trained and supervised community interventionists have shown effectiveness in Nepal and Indonesia (Tol et al., 2010; Jordans et al., 2010). The interventions reduced psycho-social difficulties and aggression among boys and increased pro-social behaviors in girls but did not result in a reduction of PTSD symptoms, anxiety, or depression (Jordans et al., 2010). The investigators concluded that this type of intervention should be implemented in conjunction with more targeted specialist services for affected children.

This was done in a three-tier program in Bosnia (Layne et al., 2008): the tier 1 intervention included school-based psycho-education and skills training and was effective at significantly reducing PTSD and depressive symptoms. The tier 2 intervention included both classroom intervention as well as a seventeen-session manual-based group and found greater improvements for PTSD and depressive symptoms as well as improvements in maladaptive grief. A small number of very distressed students with acute risk of self-harm were referred to community specialist services (tier 3). The three-tier approach made efficient use of a variety of skill levels. The study took place in a middle-income country where specialist CAMHS were available.

In recent years the focus in some studies has broadened beyond PTSD symptomatology to include a wider variety of both psychiatric symptoms (e.g., anxiety or depression) and indicators of general well-being (e.g., a sense of hope or coping skills). Studies also increasingly examine gender-specific responses to treatment with some studies showing greater effectiveness in girls (e.g., Tol, 2010) and others in boys (e.g., Qouta et al., 2012); the mechanisms for these differential effects are being assessed. Furthermore, researchers focus more on the moderating role of vulnerability and protective factors on the intervention's effectiveness and increasingly take an ecological view involving social systems such as families, schools, and community centers in the treatments (Qouta et al., 2012; Tol et al., 2012; Wolmer et al., 2011).

Table 6.2. Trauma-related disorders

Setting	*Study Design*	*Sample*	*Intervention*	*Comparison group*	*Main results*
Kosovo (Gordon, 2008)	RCT, three-month follow-up	Eighty-two adolescents meeting criteria for PTSD	Twelve-session mind-body group program by high school teachers	waitlist	Significantly lower PTSD scores following the intervention than control group ($p < .001$) maintained at follow-up. After the wait-list control group received the intervention, there was a significant decrease ($p < .001$) in PTSD scores compared to preintervention.
Ten schools in central Bosnia (Layne, 2008)	RCT, four-month follow-up	127 children with severe symptoms of PTSD, depression, or maladaptive grief	Three-tiered program with psycho-education (tier 1), classroom/ community-based interventions (tier 2), and CAMHS (tier 3)	Psycho-education (tier 1) only	Significant ($p < .05$) reductions in PTSD symptoms (58% at posttreatment, 81% at follow-up), depression symptoms (23% at posttreatment, 61% at follow-up) and maladaptive grief reactions were found in the treatment condition.
Gaza, Palestine (Qouta 2012)	RCT	Ten- to thirteen-year-old war-affected schoolchildren	School-based intervention using teaching recovery techniques (TRT) during sixteen sessions	Usual school-provided support	intervention effectiveness were specific to gender and peritraumatic dissociation. At T2, the intervention significantly reduced the proportion of clinical PTSS among boys, and both the symptom level ($R(2) = .24$), and proportion of clinical PTSS among girls who had a low level of peritraumatic dissociation.

Refugee camp in Northeast Sri Lanka (Catani, 2009)	RCT, six month follow-up	Thirty-one children with tsunami-induced PTSD	Narrative Exposure Therapy for children (KIDNET) in six sessions	meditation-relaxation (MED-RELAX) sessions	At six months follow-up, recovery rates were 81% for the children in the KIDNET group and 71% for those in the MED-RELAX group. There was no significant difference between the two therapy groups in any outcome measure.
Sri Lanka (Tol, 2012)	RCT	399 war-affected children	Fifteen manualized sessions over five weeks of cognitive behavioral techniques and creative expressive elements	waitlist	No significant overall effects on PTSD, depressive, or anxiety symptoms. A main effect in favor of intervention was for conduct problems, especially for younger children. Boys and children experiencing lower levels of current war-related stressors showed stronger effects on PTSD, anxiety, and function impairment.
Central Sulawesi, Indonesia (Tol, 2010)	cluster RCT, follow-up	403 children aged eight to thirteen with PTSD and anxiety symptoms	School-based psychosocial intervention combining CTG and creative expressive techniques	waitlist	Intervention showed maintained hope ($p = .001$), increased positive coping ($p = .015$), maintained peer social support ($p < .001$), and increased play social support ($p < .001$). Girls showed larger treatment benefits on PTSD symptoms ($p <= .004$).
Rural Nepal (Jordans, 2010)	cluster RCT	325 children aged eleven to fourteen with elevated psychosocial distress	School-based intervention	no intervention	After correcting no evidence for treatment effects was found on any outcome variable. Additional analyses showed gender effects for treatment on prosocial behavior (2.70), psychological difficulties (-2.19), and aggression (-4.42).

(continued)

Table 6.2. *(Continued)*

Setting	*Study Design*	*Sample*	*Intervention*	*Comparison group*	*Main results*
Afghanistan (Kalantari, 2012)	RCT	Eighty-eight war-bereaved Afghani refugees, aged twelve to eighteen years	"Writing for Recovery" group intervention is a new treatment approach developed by the Children and War Foundation	no intervention	The difference of Traumatic Grief Inventory for Children (TGIC) scores between the experimental group in pretest and posttest was significant ($p = .001$). Results of analysis of covariance also showed a significant effect of Writing for Recovery on the experimental group ($p < .001$).
Conflict-affected communities in Poso, Indonesia (Tol, 2008)	cluster RCT	495 children aged eight to thirteen with PTSD and anxiety symptoms	School-based psychosocial intervention combining CBT and creative expressive techniques	no intervention	Significantly more improvement in posttraumatic stress disorder symptoms (2.78) and maintained hope (-2.21) in the treatment group than control group. No group difference was seen in changes in stress-related physical symptoms (0.50), depressive symptoms (0.70), anxiety (0.12), or functioning (0.52).
Rwanda (Schaal, 2009)	RCT, follow-up six months	Twenty-six genocide orphans who presented with PTSD	individual narrative exposure therapy (NET)	group interpersonal psychotherapy (IPT)	At post-test, there were no significant group differences between NET and IPT on outcome measures. However there was a significant time x treatment interaction in PTSD (p < .05) and depression symptoms (p= .05). At follow-up, NET participants were significantly more improved than IPT (25% fulfill PTSD criteria versus 71%) with respect to both the severity of symptoms of PTSD and depression.

Two refugee camps in Northern Uganda (Bolton, 2007)	RCT	314 adolescents aged fourteen to seventeen years from refugee camps	group interpersonal psychotherapy intervention or creative play intervention during sixteen weeks	waitlist	Group IPT reduced depression symptoms with a mean difference in change of 9.79 (girls 12.61, boys not significant 5.72) in survivors of war and displacement in Uganda, while creative workshops showed no effect (-2.51).
Southwestern Uganda (Kumakech, 2009)	cluster RCT, ten week follow-up	326 AIDS orphans aged ten to fifteen years	school-based peer-group support intervention	no intervention	The intervention showed significant improvement in depression ($p< .001$), anger ($p< .0001$), and anxiety ($p= .003$), but not for self-concept $p= .24$) as supposed to the control group.
Refugee camp in Northern Uganda (Ertl, 2011)	RCT follow-up one year	85 former child soldiers with PTSD aged twelve to twenty-five years	narrative exposure therapy (NET) in eight sessions by trained local lay therapists or an academic catch-up program	waitlist	NET produced a larger within-treatment effect size (Cohen $d= 1.80$) than academic catch-up ($d= .83$) and waitlisting ($d= .81$).
Northern Uganda (Betancourt, 2012)	RCT	304 displaced war-affected children with significant depression symptoms	Interpersonal Psychotherapy Group (IPT-G)	Play/recreation group or wait-list	IPT-G brought most effect among female subjects without an abdcution history (E =1.06). IPT-G was effective for treatment of depression for both male and female subjects with a history of abdcution (E = .92 and .50).

The settings and types of trauma the affected children have been directly or indirectly exposed to vary widely. They range from former Ugandan child soldiers still living in unstable conditions who have been exposed to extreme violence often involving torture, forced participation in atrocities, sexual violence, and the loss of loved ones (Ertl et al., 2011), to studies in relatively settled communities after natural disasters or once war has subsided (e.g., Layne et al., 2008).

Evidence from HIC

Evidence from HIC might be of limited use as it often focuses on single traumatic events (such as a car accident or rape), or on individuals exposed to more chronic trauma (such as child abuse), with only limited work on more comparable larger traumatic events such as natural or manmade disasters. The therapeutic modalities mentioned above, such as CBT, IPT, NET as well as relaxation techniques and in recent times eye movement desensitization and reprocessing (EMDR), have all been used with positive effects, but none have sufficient evidence in use with children to warrant a 1a rating of their evidence level (Yule, 2008).

Implications for Practice in LAMIC

It is encouraging to see increasing evidence that children exposed to war, disaster and other traumas can be effectively treated in low-resource settings even if they still live in insecure circumstances or refugee camps and even if the exposure has been extreme. Qualitative studies carried out prior to the interventions have proven to be extremely important at identifying local idioms of distress, culturally appropriate and acceptable interventions, and available local support systems. Offering a multi-tiered approach makes sense as it uses scarce resources well, ensuring that children receive the right level of care appropriate to their needs. However, they do depend on the presence of some form of specialist service. All RCTs have used programs specifically adapted to be cost effective and feasible. Given the frequent lack of exact diagnoses, the diversity of interventions, settings and nature of the traumatic events as well as the generally short-term follow-up, it is too early to say exactly what works for whom and when; however, the evidence base is improving

Managing Developmental Disorders Including Autism

Introduction

"Developmental disorders" (DD) is the umbrella term used by mhGAP to describe a variety of problems including mental retardation and intellectual disability (ID) as well as autism spectrum disorders (ASD). These disorders are chronic, usually have childhood onset, and persist in a steady course into adulthood. In LAMIC DD can also be the consequence of malnutrition or disease (most notably cerebral malaria and HIV/AIDS), and accurate diagnosis is often unavailable. Interventions are usually not aimed at cure but either at preventing or managing the disorder by increasing independence and access to community resources. Left untreated and with no services available in LAMI settings these children are often isolated, and if they are prone to dangerous behaviors families sometimes see no choice but to physically restrain them.

Evidence from LAMIC

We found ten RCTs and a larger number of non-controlled interventions addressing the needs of children with DD. There is also a series of excellent reviews focusing on interventions aimed at parents (Einfeld et al., 2012), community-based rehabilitation (Robertson et al., 2012), and interventions for pervasive developmental disorders (Hastings et al., 2012) which include not only RCTs but other studies and personal communications with organizations dealing with intellectual disability in various parts of the world. One of the difficulties reviewing this area is that it is not always clear whether studies address intellectual, psychiatric, or physical disabilities. In the case of organic disorders such as HIV or cerebral malaria, children may have both somatic and mental health problems. In table 6.3, we focus on the psychiatric end of the spectrum excluding studies related to known physical causes (e.g., cerebral malaria, HIV, epilepsy, malnutrition or low birth weight).

The nature of the interventions varied. Many focus on working with parents, sometimes using specific packages such as the Portage curriculum in Vietnam, which brought significant improvement in most domains of adaptive behavior , personal care, and motor skills to children with ID (Shin et al., 2009). Also promising were programs training parents to deliver child-stimulating and interactive interventions at home, ranging from general activities to promote development (Potterton et al., 2010) to more specific methods such as Thai massage (Piravej et al., 2009). Psycho-education for parents and direct community support aimed at changing parental and community attitudes and skills also showed positive effects (Russell, 1999). In contrast, computerized cognitive rehabilitation training (CCRT) (e.g., Bangirana et al., 2011), which was mainly used for children with ID related to somatic causes, only found improvement on the computer tasks without generalization of effects to normal life situations. Among the biological interventions a placebo controlled RCT from India found a herbal remedy (Mentat) was effective in reducing

Table 6.3. Childhood disability and developmental disorders

Setting	*Study design*	*Sample*	*Intervention*	*Comparison group*	*Main results*
Turkey (Miral, 2007)	RCT	Thirty children aged eight to eighteen with autistic disorder	treatment with Risperidone	treatment with haloperidol	With Risperidone significantly greater reduction in the Aberrant Behavior Checklist and Turkey DSM-IV Pervasive Developmental Disorder scale scores ($P < 0.05$ and $P < 0.01$). Ritvo-Freeman Real Life Rating Scale sensory motor and language subscores decreased in the risperidone group further than the holoperidol group ($P < 0.05$).
India (Dave, 1993)	RCT	Forty children with ID and nineteen with ID and epilepsy	herbal remedy (Mentat)	placebo	Effective reduction in rating score on the Children's Behavioural Inventory test in children with mental retardation with and without epilepsy ($p < .001$).
Southern India (Russel, 1999)	RCT	Fifty-seven parents of intellectually disabled children	family psychoeducation in ten weeks	treatment as usual	Increase in parental attitude score ($p = .001$), orientation towards child-rearing skills ($p = .005$) knowledge toward intellectual disability ($p = .01$) and attitude toward management of intellectual disability ($p = .003$), but no change in attitude toward the intellectual disability subscale ($p = .06$).

Vietnam (Shin, 2009)	RCT	Thirty-seven children aged three to six with intellectual disabilities (ID)	home-based one-year intervention based on Portage Curriculum consisting of training and coaching of parents	no intervention	Intervention group improved significantly in most domains of the Vineland Adaptive Behavior Scales ($p< .05$), and also performed significantly better than the control group in the areas of personal care ($p< .05$) and motor skills ($p< .05$).
Red Cross Center in Thailand (Piravej, 2009)	RCT	Sixty autistic children between the ages of three and ten	Thai Traditional Massage (TTM) in addition to sensory integration	treatment as usual (sensory integration)	The Connors' Parent Questionnaire detected only improvement for anxiety ($p = .04$) in the massage group, whereas when both groups were compared, a significant improvement in conduct problem ($p = .03$) and anxiety ($p = .01$) was found.
Thailand (Sampanthavivat, 2012)	RCT	Sixty children aged three to nine with autistic disorder	Twenty sessions of hyperbaric oxygen treatment (HBOT)	placebo treatment with sham air	Autism Treatment Evaluation Checklist score (ATEC) significantly improved after intervention in both arms ($P < 0.001$ in both groups by parents, $P = 0.015$ in HBOT group and $P = 0.004$ in sham group by clinician) with no significant difference between groups.

behavioral and cognitive deficits in children with mental retardation both with and without epilepsy (Dave et al., 1993); risperidone also improved some aspects of behavior in Turkish children with DD more than haloperidol (Miral et al., 2008). Hyperbaric oxygen showed no effects compared to a control group treated with sham air, but both groups showed significant overall improvement (Sampanthavivat et al., 2012).

Much more evidence is available from evaluations (mostly non-RCTs) of the WHO Community Rehabilitation Programme (CBP) which is highly effective in helping disabled children to become more independent, take up schooling, and increase social inclusion.

Evidence from HIC

A number of behavioral interventions, mainly delivered by parents, as well as psychopharmacological interventions and educational programs, show some level of effectiveness, but none reach the 1a level of evidence. Some of the associated features of autism spectrum disorders can be effectively managed with medication such as antipsychotics (especially risperidone and aripiprazol) for aggression and stimulants for hyperactivity (Rowels et al., 2012).

Implications for Practice in LAMIC

Even though rigorous RCTs are scarce, many reports show the WHO CBR approach can be highly effective in increasing disabled people's independence, improving access to school and work, and improving parents' and communities' attitudes toward disability; however, it needs to extend more to psychiatric and intellectual disabilities (Robertson et al., 2012). It is uncertain at this stage whether children would benefit from a more specific treatment approach and to what extent early intervention and stimulation might improve long-term outcomes further (see also under "Preventive Interventions" below). As behavioral problems often co-exist with (pervasive) developmental disorders, and pose the largest burden on families, parent management training is highly recommended for further implementation and research (Hastings et al., 2012; Mejia, 2012).

Depressive and/or Anxiety Symptoms (Including Somatisation and Obsessive Compulsive Disorder)

Introduction

The prevalence of depression and anxiety disorders rises sharply in adolescence, particularly in girls, who are 1.5–3 times more likely to develop depression than boys. Both major disorders, as well as subclinical symptoms of depression and anxiety, occur worldwide and have great public health implications. Depression increases risk of suicide which is a major cause of death particularly in young women in India and China.

Evidence from LAMIC

Outside the context of trauma we found only one completed RCT (Tang et al., 2009) for treating depressive disorders exclusively among adolescents, and two trials targeting school children with subclinical depression. An RCT using intensive IPT delivered by fully trained school counselors and psychology interns achieved significantly reduced depression symptoms in a sample of depressed adolescents with suicidal risk and para-suicidal behavior (Tang et al., 2009). An RCT carried out in China using the PennOptimism program, based on CBT principles, on 220 subclinically depressed school children showed a significant reduction in depressive symptoms in the intervention group post-treatment and at the three- and six-month follow-ups (Yu, 2002).

A number of RCTs assessed the efficacy of psychological treatments for depression in LAMIC in adults, some of which included young people from the age of sixteen years. The most effective approaches were community treatments using group IPT techniques in Uganda (Bass et al., 2006; Bolton et al., 2003) or multi-component stepped-care approaches in Chile ranging from psycho education for the least affected to pharmacotherapy for the most severely affected (Araya et al., 2003).

Most Robust Evidence from HIC

The psychological therapies CBT and IPT have the most robust record of effectiveness for depression with no significant difference between the two methods (Schloredt et al., 2008). For anxiety disorders and obsessive compulsive disorders (OCD), CBT has the best evidence base. It can be delivered individually, in a group or family. For the under-eleven age group especially, involvement of parents is helpful. Pharmacotherapy has also been evaluated for anxiety and depressive disorders in young people. For moderate to severe anxiety and depressive disorders, SSRIs have shown effectiveness. Fluoxetine has the safest risk/benefit balance and produces significant improvement in clinical symptoms and improved likelihood of remission for depression. Reviews show tricyclic antidepressants are ineffective for depression in children and adolescents (Brent, 2008). SSRIs and clomipramine are more effective than placebo in the treatment of OCD. For other anxiety disorders and other medications, such as benzodiazepines, 5-HT agonists, and tricyclics, there is insufficient evidence for usefulness in anxious children and adolescents (Brent, 2008; Schloredt et al., 2008).

Implications for Practice in LAMIC

Given the enormous health burden of depressive disorders and associated adolescent suicides in many LAMIC, it is surprising that so few studies have addressed this problem. In China, IPT therapists are being trained to a high standard to deliver effective and acceptable treatment so these techniques seem to be transculturally adaptable. In trauma treatment a number of low-cost, feasible interventions (both group and individual) building on the principles of the most effective psychological treatments developed in HIC (IPT and CBT) have reduced symptoms of anxiety and depression. Structuring daily activities as well as keeping physically fit are strategies regularly linked to positive outcomes mirroring results from HIC (Bonhauser et al., 2005). Further dissemination and testing on larger samples and clinical groups is required.

PREVENTIVE INTERVENTIONS

Optimizing Childhood Development

Evidence from LAMIC

Many studies have tested interventions in the 0–3 year age group with the aim of promoting neuro-cognitive functioning throughout life. These include nutritional supplements as well as cognitive stimulation programs. We found almost sixty RCTs showing that various nutritional supplements, especially iodine, iron, fatty acids, and some micronutrients, have led to cognitive function gains (details available from the authors).

In a review of fifty-three studies using low-cost but resource-intensive child stimulation programs carried out by mothers of young children, sixteen came from LAMIC (Maulik, 2009). Typically mothers are taught to play with their children, read to them, praise them, and give them positive reinforcement. Sometimes toys and picture books are provided; sometimes specific methods such as baby massage or music are used. Stimulation through play and reading were effective, and stimulation through music and massage was promising. In one such study from Jamaica which combined dietary supplements with early stimulation benefits were maintained into adolescence with the intervention group showing fewer symptoms of depression and anxiety, less suspension from school, better attention span, reductions in problem and violent behavior, and better self-esteem (Walker et al., 2011; Walker et al., 2010;

Walker et al., 2006). Early stimulation combined with nutritional supplements worked better than supplements alone. Kangaroo Mother Care is a specific program for low birth weight and pre-term babies which has been successfully adapted to low resource settings (Maulik, 2009; Tessier et al., 2009). Cooper et al. (2009) focused particularly on the mother-infant relationship to promote sensitive and responsive parenting and secure attachment from infant to mother which is known to be a strong protective factor predicting favorable child development. The intervention was delivered by local lay women and had a significant positive impact not only on the infant-mother relationship and their attachment but also on mother's depressed mood six months postintervention. Further evidence for the effectiveness of early stimulation comes from a longitudinal epidemiological study from Brazil (Barros et al., 2010). Interestingly the effect of stimulation was particularly strong among mothers with low schooling.

Most Robust Evidence from HIC

Many of the programs used in LAMIC have been developed in HIC as public health programs for disadvantaged groups. Some, like "Head Start," have been scaled up to national programs. Effect sizes were usually higher in initial small-scale RCTs compared to interventions delivered to whole populations and maintaining program fidelity is an issue to be considered in wide scale dissemination (Medicine NRCaIo, 2009).

Implications for Practice in LAMIC

Even though interventions are quite diverse, numbers sometimes small, and research designs not always rigorous, there is quite strong evidence that early stimulation, especially through play, reading, and sensitive responsive parenting, can significantly improve cognitive development and decrease behavioral problems. Epidemiological data suggest that effects are particularly high in mothers with low schooling.

Preventing Risk-Taking Behaviors in Adolescence

Evidence from LAMIC

Many studies, some of them large-scale, were carried out to reduce risk-taking behavior in adolescence including preventing drug and alcohol abuse. Usually studies found large increases in knowledge, improved attitudes, and educational planning within the intervention groups, but often follow-up periods were too short to find actual reductions in HIV infection rates and other biological markers (Dick, 2006; Cowan et al., 2010; Doyle et al., 2010).

DISCUSSION

How Can We Use the Available Evidence to Develop Child Mental Health Interventions?

The evidence presented in this paper is pioneering and impressive in many ways but still far too limited to give a definitive answer to the question "what works where?" Carrying out more and better designed RCTs takes many years. Evidence-based (level 1a) child mental health interventions are often complex and expensive, requiring years of training in specific (often copyrighted or protected) treatment packages. Despite limitations in the evidence a number of principles have been established for providing CAMH interventions in LAMIC (Kieling et al., 2011; Patel, 2007a; Patel, 2007b; De Jong, 2002; Eisenbruch, 2004). Many of the successful programs referred to here have used a stepwise approach when designing an intervention in LAMIC. Steps differed slightly but generally included the following elements.

Step 1: Assess needs in interaction with beneficiaries.

For this exploratory step a mixed method model is often recommended. Qualitative methods achieve a better understanding of the local explanatory models of disease (Kleinman, 1989), local idioms of distress, societal strengths such as existing support systems, beneficial child rearing practices, locally available resources, and general acceptability as well as barriers to treatment. Locally available epidemiological data including data from local health centers, papers in languages other than English, or unpublished reports (if available) can all contribute to this exploratory phase.

Step 2: Identify and prioritize intervention modalities that could address these needs.

Evidence from HIC reviews like this one or the PLoS series (Lund et al., 2012) can help identify the most promising interventions for various settings.

Step 3: Strip down or unpack the intervention modalities to identify the evidence-based elements of sometimes complex treatments, and simplify to make them affordable.

The reviewed studies show it is possible to strip down some of the often complex and expensive interventions developed in HIC to basic principles and successfully train lay community members to deliver them. We must, however, be aware of the danger of program drift as diluting interventions too much can lead them to become ineffective.

Step 4: Use evidence-based treatment elements to design treatment packages that are acceptable and sustainable locally.

For this step results from the qualitative first phase are combined with the results from steps two and three. To be acceptable and sustainable treatment packages need to use local resources, local idioms of distress, and local strength, and they need to be delivered locally where they are needed. Even the most cost-effective programs require on-going funding and support, and one of the problems noted in this review was that many studies had no or very short follow-up periods which might mean that interventions stop being delivered at the end of the initial funding period. Especially in the field of child mental health, there is much discussion on where services can best be embedded (e.g., schools, primary health care, primary mental health care, social care, etc.), and solutions will vary locally.

Step 5: Assess intervention acceptability and effectiveness, and be willing to adjust programs if they appear to be unacceptable or not working.

It might appear a waste of resources to spend large amounts on research and evaluation instead of patient care; however, in contexts of scarcity it is even less responsible to waste resources on interventions that do not work. The careful evaluation of programs benefits people locally and adds to global knowledge.

What Are the Most Promising Treatment Components Coming out of This Review?

There is strong evidence that young children all over the world benefit cognitively, emotionally, and behaviorally when adults stimulate them through regular positive attention and play and sensitively respond to their needs; these benefits seem to extend into adolescence.

Children with disruptive disorders appear to benefit from parenting approaches aimed at positively reinforcing desired behavior and firm but consistent non-violent boundary setting. While child-rearing practices in most societies include elements of these principles parents and teachers across the world seem capable of learn to apply them better and more consistently. The delivery mode and emphasis put on various elements of the training might need careful adaptation to cultural needs and sensitivities, but research suggests that both children and their parents can benefit from the interventions.

There is also strong evidence that many severely traumatized children can be helped through treatment. Tiered approaches with psychoeducation and skills training for some and more intensive treatments for others make best use of available resources. Specialist services are needed to support community-based treatments and cater for the most severely affected youngsters. Currently there is insufficient evidence to support any one particular form of therapy, and gender-differentiated treatment response is not yet fully understood. Again, emphasis should be put on what is acceptable and possibly already available in communities, and one package might not suit all.

Adolescence is a particularly vulnerable time in terms of mental health and is associated with increased prevalence of anxiety and depressive disorders. For such common mental disorders, treatment principles derived from CBT and IPT as well as some risk-prevention strategies seem to be effective across many cultures.

LIMITATIONS OF THIS REVIEW

Firstly, considering LAMIC as if it was one entity does not do justice to the great diversity of economic, cultural, and social environments involved. There is uncertainty about whether interventions that work in European or Arab communities can translate unaltered to African societies, Brazilian favelas, or Asian refugee camps. We are very aware of this limitation and have discussed ways to make interventions culturally appropriate above.

The second limitation is the low to moderate standard of trials compared to trials in HIC. Through lack of diagnostic capacity the exact nature of the disorders treated is often unknown, and the follow-up period short or non-existent. The use of lay therapists might work well with close supervision but can lead to lack of therapeutic fidelity over longer follow-up. We considered applying the GRADE (Grading of Recommendations, Assessment, Development, and Evaluation) software (Guyatt et al., 2011) but found only a handful of studies gave the necessary information on blinding, concealment of randomization, etc., so in the end we refrained from the exercise.

Thirdly, there is much information available outside the scope of this chapter but which might, nonetheless, be helpful to those trying to set up interventions in low-resource areas (non-RCT trials, studies published in languages other than English, etc.). For some specific disorders and regions much more detailed information is available, and we have included some of the references in this review.

Finally, the sorting and presenting of the information was led by the studies already available. Where possible we sorted them by classification systems used by WHOs mhGAP. In other cases, such as "trauma," we created a new category corresponding to practical needs as well as the relatively large body of evidence already available in the field. Other ordering systems are equally valid and feasible.

CONCLUSION

This systematic review of RCTs for child mental health interventions in LAMIC shows that many basic treatment principles developed and tested in HIC can be, and have been, successfully adapted to low-resource settings where they have brought real benefits to troubled children and their families. As a result of such interventions children have experienced less stigmatization and exclusion, have been able to attend school regularly, were able to build up hope and self-esteem in the face of disaster, and, in the case of the Ugandan child soldiers, were even able to rebuild their lives after exposure to some of the most severe and traumatic violence imaginable. Unfortunately these treatments are available to only a tiny minority of affected children.

Based on the studies and suggestions from adult mental health we developed a stepwise approach that might help in developing future interventions and make a first attempt at identifying the basic treatment elements regarding child mental health that might work in a variety of social and cultural settings.

We hope that this selective report on what works where in child mental health in LAMIC will be superseded by a larger body of work and more rigorous research evidence from diverse cultures and settings.

ACKNOWLEDGMENTS

We are grateful to the Centre for Global Mental Health at the Institute of Psychiatry in London for their support and to our employers at De Jutters for giving us the time to do this work, for which no grants or subsidies were received and no interests are declared.

REFERENCES

Araya, R., Rojas, G., Fritsch, R., Gaete, J., Rojas M., Simon, G., Peters, T. J. Treating depression in primary care in low-income women in Santiago, Chile: A randomized controlled trial. *The Lancet* 361 (2003):995–1000, doi: 10.1016/S0140-6736(03)12825-5

Baker-Henningham, H., Scott, S., Jones, K., Walker, S. Reducing child conduct problems and promoting social skills in a middle-income country: Cluster randomized controlled trial. *The British Journal of Psychiatry* 201 (2012):101–8.

Baker-Henningham, H., Walker, S., Powell, C., Gardner, J. M. Preventing behavior problems through a universal intervention in Jamaican basic schools: A pilot study. *West Indian Medical Journa*l 58 (2009a):460–64.

Baker-Henningham, H., Walker, S., Powell, C., Gardner, J. M. A pilot study of the Incredible Years Teacher Training program and a curriculum unit on social and emotional skills in community pre-schools in Jamaica. *Child Care Health and Development* 35 (2009b):624–31, doi: 10.1111/j.1365-2214.2009.00964.*x*.

Bangirana, P., Allebeck, P., Boivin, M.J., John, C.C., Page, C., Ehnvall, A., Musisi, S. Cognition, behavior, and academic skills after cognitive rehabilitation in Ugandan children surviving severe malaria: A randomized trial. *BMC Neurology* 11 (2011):96, doi: 10.1186/1471-2377-11-96.

Barlow, J., Coren, E., Stewart-Brown, S. Parent-training programs for improving maternal psychosocial health. *Cochrane Database of Systematic Reviews* (2004), doi: 10.1002/14651858.CD002020.pub2.

Bass, J., Neugebauer, R., Clougherty, K. F., Verdeli, H., Wickramartne, P., Ngodoni, L., Speelman, L., Weissman, M., Bolton, P. Group interpersonal psychotherapy for depression in rural Uganda: 6-month outcomes: randomized controlled trial. *British Journal of Psychiatry* 188 (2006):567–73, doi: 10.1192/bjp.188.6.567.

Berger, R., Gelkopf, M. School-based intervention for the treatment of tsunami-related distress in children: A quasi-randomized controlled trial. *Psychotherapy and Psychosomatics* 78 (2009):364–71, doi: 10.1159/000235976.

Betancourt, T. S., et al. Moderators of treatment effectiveness for war-affected youth with depression in northern Uganda. *Journal of Adolescent Health* 51.6 (2012):544–50.

Bolton, P., Bass, J., Betancourt, T., Speelman, L., Onyango, G., Clougherty, K. F., Neugebauer, R., Murray, L., Verdeli, H. Interventions for depression symptoms among adolescent survivors of war and displacement in northern Uganda: A randomized controlled trial. *JAMA—Journal of the American Medical Association* 298 (2007):519–27, doi: 10.1001/jama.298.5.519.

Bolton, P., Bass, J., Neugebauer, R., Verdeli, H., et al. Group interpersonal psychotherapy for depression in rural Uganda: A randomized controlled trial. *JAMA—Journal of the American Medical Association* 289 (2003):3117–24, doi: 10.1001/jama.289.23.3117.

Bonhauser, M., Fernandez, G., Püschel, K., Yanez, F., Montero, J, Thompson, B., Coronado, G. Improving physical fitness and emotional well-being in adolescents of low socioeconomic status in Chile: Results of a school-based controlled trial. *Health Promotion International* 20 (2005):113–22, doi: 10.1093/heapro/dah603.

Brent, D., Weersing, V. Depressive disorders in childhood and adolescence. In Rutter, M., Bishop, D., Pine, D., et al. (Eds.), *Rutter's Child and Adolescent Psychiatry*. Oxford: Blackwell Publishing Ltd., 2008.

Catani C., Kohiladevy, M., Ruf, M., Schauer, E., Elbert, T., Neuner, F. Treating children traumatized by war and Tsunami: A comparison between exposure therapy and meditation-relaxation in North-East Sri Lanka. *BMC Psychiatry* 9 (2009):22, doi: 10.1186/1471-244X-9-22.

CEMB: Centre of Evidence Based Medicine. Levels of Evidence (March 2009). Accessed on August 25, 2013, http://www.cebm.net/index.aspx?o=1025.

Collett, T. Bipolar and attention deficit hyperactivity disorder in children: An analysis of the recent literature. San Diego: Alliant International University, 2009.

Collins, P. Y., Patel, V., Joestl, S. S., et al. Grand challenges in global mental health. *Nature* 475 (2011):27–30, doi: 10.1038/475027a.

Cooper, P. J., et al. Improving quality of mother-infant relationship and infant attachment in socioeconomically deprived community in South Africa: Randomized controlled trial. *BMJ: British Medical Journal* 338 (2009):b974, doi: 10.1136/bmj.b974.

Cowan, F. M., Pascoe, S. J. S., Langhaug, L. F., Mavhu, W., Chidiya, S., Jaffar, S., Mbizvo, M. T., Stephenson, J. M., Johnson, A. M., Power, R. M., Woelk, G., Hayes, R. J. The Regai Dzive Shiri project: Results of a randomized trial of an HIV prevention intervention for youth. *AIDS* 24 (2010):2541–52, doi:10.1097/QAD.0b013e32833e77c9.

Dave, U. P., Chauvan, V., Dalvi, J. Evaluation of BR-16 A (Mentat) in cognitive and behavioral dysfunction of mentally retarded children—a placebo-controlled study. *Indian Journal of Pediatrics* 60 (1993):423–28, doi: 10.1007/BF02751207.

De Jong, J. T. V. M., Van Ommeren, M. Toward a culture-informed epidemiology: Combining qualitative and quantitative research in transcultural contexts. *Transcultural Psychiatry* 39.4 (2012):422–33.

Dick, B., Ferguson, J., Ross, D. A. Preventing HIV/AIDS in young people: A systematic review of the evidence from developing countries: Introduction and Rationale. *WHO Technical Report Series* 938 (2006):1–341.

Doyle, A. M., Ross, D. A., Maganja, K., Baisley, K., Masesa, C., et al. Long-term biological and behavioral impact of an adolescent sexual health intervention in Tanzania: Follow-up survey of the community-based MEMA kwa Vijana Trial. *PLoS Medicine* 7 (2010):e1000287, doi: 10.1371/journal.pmed.1000287.

Dybdahl, R. Children and mothers in war: an outcome study of a psychosocial intervention program. *Child Development* 72 (2001):1214–30, doi: 10.1111/1467-8624.00343.

Einfeld, S. L., et al. Interventions provided by parents for children with intellectual disabilities in low and middle income countries. *Journal of Applied Research in Intellectual Disabilities* 25.2 (2012):135–42.

Eisenbruch, M., De Jong, J., Van de Put, W. Bringing order out of chaos: A culturally competent approach to managing the problems of refugees and victims of organized violence. *Journal of Traumatic Stress* 17.2 (2004):123–31.

Ertl, V., Pfeiffer, A., Schauer, E., Elbert, T., Neuner, F. Community-implemented trauma therapy for former child soldiers in Northern Uganda: A randomized controlled trial. *JAMA-Journal of the American Medical Association* 306 (2011):503–12, doi: 10.1001/jama.2011.1060.

Gau, S. S. F., et al. A randomized, double-blind, placebo-controlled clinical trial on once-daily atomoxetine hydrochloride in Taiwanese children and adolescents with attention-deficit/hyperactivity disorder. *Journal of child and adolescent psychopharmacology* 17.4 (2007):447–60.

Gordon, J. S., Staples, J. K., Blyta, A., Bytyqi, M., Wilson, A. T. Treatment of posttraumatic stress disorder in postwar Kosovar adolescents using mind-body skills groups: A randomized controlled trial. *Journal of Clinical Psychiatry* 69 (2008):1469–76, doi: ej07m03828.

Graeff-Martins, A. S., Oswald, S., Comassetto, J. O., Kieling, C., Goncalves, R. R., Rohde, L. A. A package of interventions to reduce school dropout in public schools in a developing country: A feasibility study. *European Child and Adolescent Psychiatry* 15 (2006):442–49, doi: 10.1007/s00787-006-0555-2.

Guyatt, G., Oxman, A. D., Akl, E. A., et al. GRADE guidelines: 1. Introduction-GRADE evidence profiles and summary of findings tables. *Journal of Clinical Epidemiology* 64 (2011):383–94, doi: 10.1016/j.jclinepi.2010.04.026.

Hastings, R. P., Robertson, J., Yasamy, M. T., et al. Interventions for children with pervasive developmental disorders in low and middle income countries. *Journal of Applied Research in Intellectual Disabilities* 25.2 (2012):119–34.

Hinton, D. E., et al. A randomized controlled trial of cognitive-behavior therapy for Cambodian refugees with treatment-resistant PTSD and panic attack: A cross-over design. *Journal of traumatic stress* 18.6 (2005):617–29.

Hong, L., Yufeng, W., Agho, K., Jacobs, J. Preventing behavior problems among elementary schoolchildren: Impact of a universal school-based program in China. *Journal of School Health* 81 (2011):273–80, doi: 10.1111/j.1746-1561.2011.00592.x.

Jordans, M. J. D., et al. A controlled evaluation of a brief parenting psychoeducation intervention in Burundi. *Social psychiatry and psychiatric epidemiology* (2012):1–9.

Jordans, M. J. D., Komproe, I. H., Tol, W. A., Kohrt, B. A., Luitel, N. P., Macy, R. D., de Jong, J. T. V. M. Evaluation of a classroom-based psychosocial intervention in conflict-affected Nepal: A cluster randomized controlled trial. *Journal of Child Psychology and Psychiatry* 51 (2010):818–26, doi: 10.1111/j.1469-7610.2010.02209.x.

Kalantari, M., et al. Efficacy of writing for recovery on traumatic grief symptoms of Afghani refugee bereaved adolescents: A randomized control trial. *OMEGA—Journal of Death and Dying* 65.2 (2012):139–50.

Kieling, C., et al. Child and adolescent mental health worldwide: Evidence for action. *The Lancet* 378 (2011):1515–25.

Kleinman, A. *The illness narratives: Suffering, healing, and the human condition.* New York: Basic Books, 1989.

Kumakech, E., Cantor-Graae, E., Maling, S., Bajunirwe, F. Peer-group support intervention improves the psychosocial well-being of AIDS orphans: Cluster randomized trial. *Social Science and Medicine* 68 (2009):1038–43, doi: 10.1016/j.socscimed.2008.10.033.

Layne, C. M., Saltzman, W. R., Poppleton, L., et al. Effectiveness of a school-based group psychotherapy program for war-exposed adolescents: a randomized controlled trial. *Journal of the American Acadamy of Child and Adolescent Psychiatry* 47 (2008):1048–62, doi: 10.1097/CHI.0b013e31817eecae.

Lesmana, C. B., Suryani, L. K., Jensen, G. D., Tiliopoulos, N. A spiritual-hypnosis assisted treatment of children with PTSD after the 2002 Bali terrorist attack. *American Journal of Clinical Hypnosis* 52 (2009):23–34, doi: 10.1080/00029157.2009.10401689.

Lopez, A. D., et al. Global and regional burden of disease and risk factors, 2001: Systematic analysis of population health data. *The Lancet* 367 (2006):1747–57.

Lund, C., et al. PRIME: A program to reduce the treatment gap for mental disorders in five low-and middle-income countries. *PLoS medicine* 9 (2012):e1001359.

Martenyi, F., et al. Atomoxetine in children and adolescents with attention-deficit/hyperactivity disorder: A 6-week, randomized, placebo-controlled, double-blind trial in Russia. *European Child andAadolescent Psychiatry* 19 (2010):57–66.

Matos, M., Bauermeister, J. J., Bernal, G. Parent-child interaction therapy for Puerto Rican preschool children with ADHD and behavior problems: A pilot efficacy study. *Family Process* 48 (2009):232–52, doi: 10.1111/j.1545-5300.2009.01279.x.

Maulik, P. K., Darmstadt, G. L. Community-based interventions to optimize early childhood development in low resource settings. *Journal of Perinatology* 29 (2009):531–42, doi: 10.1038/jp.2009.42.

Medicine NRCaIo. Implementation and dissemination of prevention programs. In O'Connell, M. E., Boat, T., Warner, K. E. (Eds.), *Preventing Mental, Emotional, and Behavioral Disorders Among Young People: Progress and Possibilities*. Washington, DC: National Academies Press, 2009.

Mejia, A., Calam, R., Sanders, M. R. A review of parenting programs in developing countries: Opportunities and challenges for preventing emotional and behavioral difficulties in children. *Clinical child and family psychology review* 15.2 (2012):163–75.

Miller, T., et al. Cost-effectiveness of school support for orphan girls to prevent HIV infection in Zimbabwe. *Prevention Science* (2013):1–10.

Miral, S., et al. Risperidone versus haloperidol in children and adolescents with AD. *European Child and adolescent psychiatry* 17.1 (2008):1–8.

Nair, V., Mahadevan, S., Andomized controlled study-efficacy of clonidine versus carbamazepine in children with ADHD. *Journal of Tropical Pediatrics* 55 (2009):116–21, doi: 10.1093/tropej/fmn117.

Oveisi, S., Ardabili, H. E., Dadds, M. R., Majdzadeh, R., Mohammadkhani, P., Rad, J. A., Shahrivar, Z. Primary prevention of parent-child conflict and abuse in Iranian mothers: A randomized-controlled trial. *Child Abuse & Neglect* 34 (2010):206–13, doi: 10.1016/j.chiabu.2009.05.008.

Patel, V., Flisher A. J., Hetrick, S., McGorry, P. Mental health of young people: A global public-health challenge. *The Lancet* 369 (2007a):1302–13, doi: 10.1016/S0140-6736(07)60368-7.

Patel, V., Araya, R., Chatterjee, S. et al. Treatment and prevention of mental disorders in low-income and middle-income countries. *The Lancet* 370 (2007b):991–1005, doi: 10.1016/S0140-6736(07)61240-9.

Pelham Jr, W. E., Fabiano, G. A. Evidence-based psychosocial treatments for attention deficit/hyperactivity disorder. *Journal of Clinical Child and Adolescent Psychology* 37 (2008):184–214, doi: 10.1080/15374410701818681.

Piravej, K., Tangtronchitr, P., Chandarasiri, P., Paothong, L., Sukprasong, S. Effects of Thai traditional massage on autistic children's behavior. *Journal of Alternative and Complementary Medicine* 15 (2009):1355–61, doi: 10.1089/acm.2009.0258.

Polanczyk, G., De Lima, M. S., Horta, B. L., Biederman, J., Rohde, L. A. The worldwide prevalence of ADHD: A systematic review and metaregression analysis. *American Journal of Psychiatry* 164 (2007):942–48, doi: 10.1176/appi.ajp.164.6.942.

Potterton, J., Stewart, A., Cooper, P., Becker, P. The effect of a basic home stimulation program on the development of young children infected with HIV. *Developmental Medicine and Child Neurology* 52 (2010):547–51, doi: 10.1111/j.1469-8749.2009.03534.x.

Qouta, S. R., et al. Intervention effectiveness among war-affected children: A cluster randomized controlled trial on improving mental health. *Journal of traumatic stress* 253 (2012):288–98.

Robertson, J., et al. Efficacy of community-based rehabilitation for children with or at significant risk of intellectual disabilities in low-and middle-income countries: A review. *Journal of Applied Research in Intellectual Disabilities* 25.2 (2012):143–54.

Rowles, B. M., Hertzer, J. L. & Findling, R. L. (2012). Antipsychotic agents. In Rosenberg, D. R. & Gershon, S. (Eds.), *Pharmacotherapy of Child & Adolescent Psychiatric Disorders*. Third Edition. Oxford: Wiley-Blackwell. 181–219.

Russell, P. S., al John, J. K., Lakshmanan, J. L. Family intervention for intellectually disabled children: Randomised controlled trial. *British Journal of Psychiatry* 174 (1999):254–58, doi: 10.1192/bjp.174.3.254.

Sampanthavivat, M., et al. Hyperbaric oxygen in the treatment of childhood autism: A randomized controlled trial: Diving and hyperbaric medicine. *Journal of the South Pacific Underwater Medicine Society* 42.3 (2012):128.

Santosh, P. J., Henry, A., Varley, C. K. ADHD and hyperkinetic disorder. In Tyrer, P. J., Silk, K. R. (Eds.), *Cambridge Textbook of Effective Treatments in Psychiatry*. Cambridge: Cambridge University Press, 2008.

Schaal, S., Elbert, T., Neuner, F. (2009). Narrative exposure therapy versus interpersonal psychotherapy: A pilot randomized controlled trial with Rwandan genocide orphans. *Psychotherapy and Psychosomatics* 78 (2009):298–306, doi: 10.1159/000229768.

Schlorendt, K., Gershenson, R., Varley, C., Goodyear, I. Treatment of depressive disorders in children and adolescents. In Tyrer, P., Silk, K. (Eds.), *Cambridge Textbook of Effective Treatments in Psychiatry*. Cambridge: Cambridge University Press, 2008.

Shin, J. Y., The effects of a home-based intervention for young children with intellectual disabilities in Vietnam. *Jounal of Intellectual Disability Research* 53 (2009):339–52, doi: 10.1111/j.1365-2788.2008.01151.x.

Szobot C. M., Ketzer, C., Parente, M. A., Biederman, J., Rohde, L. A. The acute effect of methylphenidate in Brazilian male children and adolescents with ADHD: A randomized clinical trial. *Journal of Attention Disorders* 8 (2004):37–43, doi: 10.1177/108705470400800201.

Tang, T., et al. Randomized study for school-based intensive interpersonal psychotherapy for depressed adolescents with suicidal risk and parasuicide behaviors. *Psychiatry and clinical neurosciences* 63.4 (2009):463–70

Taylor, E., Sonuga-Barke, E. Disorders of attention and activity. In Rutter, M., Bishop, D. V. M., Pine, D. S., Scott, S., Stevenson, J., Taylor, E., Thapar, A. (Eds.), *Rutter's Child and Adolescent Psychiatry*. Oxford: Blackwell Publishing Ltd., 2008.

Tessier, R., Charpak, N., Giron, M., Cristo, M., de Calume, Z. F., Ruiz-Pelaez, J. G. Kangaroo mother care, home environment and father involvement in the first year of life: A randomized controlled study. *ACTA Paediatrica* 98 (2009):1444–50, doi: 10.1111/j.1651-2227.2009.01370.x.

The World Bank Group. *Country and Lending Groups*. Accessed September 9, 2011, http://data.worldbank.org/about/country-classifications/country-and-lending-groups.

Tol, W. A., Komproe, I. H., Jordans, M. J. D., Gross, A. L., Susanty, D., Macy, R. D., De Jong, J. T. V. M. Outcomes and moderators of a preventive school-based mental health intervention for children affected by war in Sri Lanka: A cluster randomized trial. *World Psychiatry* 11.2 (2012):114–22.

Tol, W. A., Komproe, I. H., Jordans, M. J. D., Gross, A. L., Susanty, D., Macy, R. D., De Jong, J. T. V. M. Mediators and moderators of a psychosocial intervention for children affected by political violence. *Journal of Consulting and Clinical Psychology* 78 (2010):818–28, doi: 10.1037/a0021348.

Tol, W. A., Komproe, I. H., Susanty, D., Macy, R. D., De Jong, J. T. V. M. School-based mental health intervention for children affected by political violence in Indonesia: A cluster randomized trial. *JAMA—Journal of the American Medical Association* 300 (2008):655–62, doi: 10.1001/jama.300-6-655.

Walker, S.P., Chang, S.M., Vera-Hernandez, M., Grantham-McGregor, S.M. "Early childhood stimulation benefits adult competence and reduces violent behavior." *Pediatrics* 127 (2011):849-57. doi: 10.1542/peds.2010-2231

Walker S. P., Chang, S. M., Younger, N., Grantham-McGregor, S. M. The effect of psychosocial stimulation on cognition and behavior at 6 years in a cohort of term, low-birthweight Jamaican children. *Developmental Medicine and Child Neurology* 52 (2010):148–54, doi: 10.1111/j.1469-8749.2010.03637.x.

Walker, S. P., Chang, S. M., Powell, C. A., Simonoff, E., Grantham-McGregor, S. M. Effects of psychosocial stimulation and dietary supplementation in early childhood on psychosocial functioning in late adolescence: Follow-up of randomized controlled trial. *British Medical Journal* 333 (2006):472, doi: 10.1136/bmj.38897.555208.2F.

WHO, War Trauma Foundation and World Vision International. (2011). *Psychological First Aid;* Guide for field workers

Wolmer, L. et al. Teacher-delivered resilience-focused intervention in schools with traumatized children following the second Lebanon war. *Journal of Traumatic Stress* 24.3 (2011):309–16.

Woolfenden, S. R., Williams, K., Peat, J. Family and parenting interventions in children and adolescents with conduct disorder and delinquency aged 10–17. *Cochrane Database of Systematic Reviews* 2 (2001):1469–93.

Yu, D. L., Seligman, M. E. P. Preventing depressive symptoms in Chinese children. *Preventive Treatment* 5 (2002):9, doi: 10.1037/1522-3736.5.1.59a.

Yule, W., Smith, P. Post-traumatic stress disorder. In Rutter M., Bishop, D. V. M., Pine, D. S., Scott, S., Stevenson, J., Taylor, E., Thapar, A. *Rutter's Child and Adolescent Psychiatry*. Oxford: Blackwell Publishing Ltd., 2008.

7

Addressing the Consequences of Violence and Adversity

The Development of a Group Mental Health Intervention for War-Affected Youth in Sierra Leone

Theresa S. Betancourt, Elizabeth A. Newnham, Katrina Hann, Ryan K. McBain, Adeyinka M. Akinsulure-Smith, John Weisz, Grace M. Lilienthal, and Nathan Hansen

It is estimated that over one billion children and adolescents live in regions affected by armed conflict (Jacob et al., 2007). Whereas access to mental health care is already very limited in low- and middle-income countries (LAMIC)—the World Health Organization (WHO) estimates the level of untreated mental disorders among adults in low- and middle-income countries may be as high as 78 percent (Kohn, Saxena, Levav & Saraceno, 2004)—the gap between the need for services and their limited availability is accentuated in regions affected by armed conflict (Betancourt, McBain, Newnham & Brennan, 2013; IASC, 2007; Walker et al., 2011). Among adolescents and youth exposed to war, psychological distress may be expressed in higher rates of internalizing problems such as PTSD, depression, withdrawal, and social isolation as well as externalizing problems (e.g., aggression, hostility) (Betancourt et al., 2013; Bryant, 2006; Johnson et al., 2008). Although many war-affected youth demonstrate great resilience, those who continue to suffer elevated levels of distress and impairment in the post-conflict environment are at risk for poor health and development, low rates of school completion, and poor economic self-sufficiency (Bayer, Klasen & Adam, 2007; Betancourt et al., 2008; Derluyn, Broekaert, Schuyten & De Temmerman, 2004). Few evidence-based interventions exist to address mental health problems in war-affected youth (Tol et al., 2011), and even fewer interventions focus on helping war-affected youth struggling with distress and impairment to navigate successful transitions to school and employment programs.

Given years of sustained exposure to violence and subsequent poly-victimization and loss among young people in war zones, it is important that the scope of interventions be broadened beyond models targeting a singular disorder such as depression or PTSD to anticipate comorbidity and diverse manifestations of complex trauma (Cloitre, 2009; Lanktree et al., in press; Peltonen & Punamäki, 2010). The present study used a multi-phase mixed methods design (see figure 7.1) to inform the development of a feasible and acceptable intervention for war-affected youth. In this design, results of a prior longitudinal study and new qualitative data were integrated to identify the focal points for intervention development. The quantitative data investigated the longitudinal trajectories of psychological distress in the post-conflict setting, and qualitative data were collected to assess specific areas of priority per the opinions of stakeholders on ongoing emotional and behavioral problems that pose obstacles to successful functioning among some war-affected youth. These findings were used to identify important intervention components and modalities for treatment delivery.

A MIXED METHODS APPROACH TO INTERVENTION DEVELOPMENT

In 2010 the team launched a new phase in a multi-phase longitudinal research project to design and evaluate a mental health intervention for war-affected youth. Intervention development built upon the evidence base being assembled via an ongoing longitudinal study of war-affected youth which has been conducted in Sierra Leone since the end of the brutal eleven-year civil war in 2002. To further root this process in the present post-conflict realities of the setting, we used mixed-methods data collection to understand the challenges facing war-affected youth in post-conflict Sierra Leone and learn from experts working with troubled youth about the core problem areas and treatment components they deemed a priority.

PRELIMINARY EVIDENCE

Our intervention development efforts in post-conflict Sierra Leone originate from a ten-year Longitudinal Study of War-Affected Youth

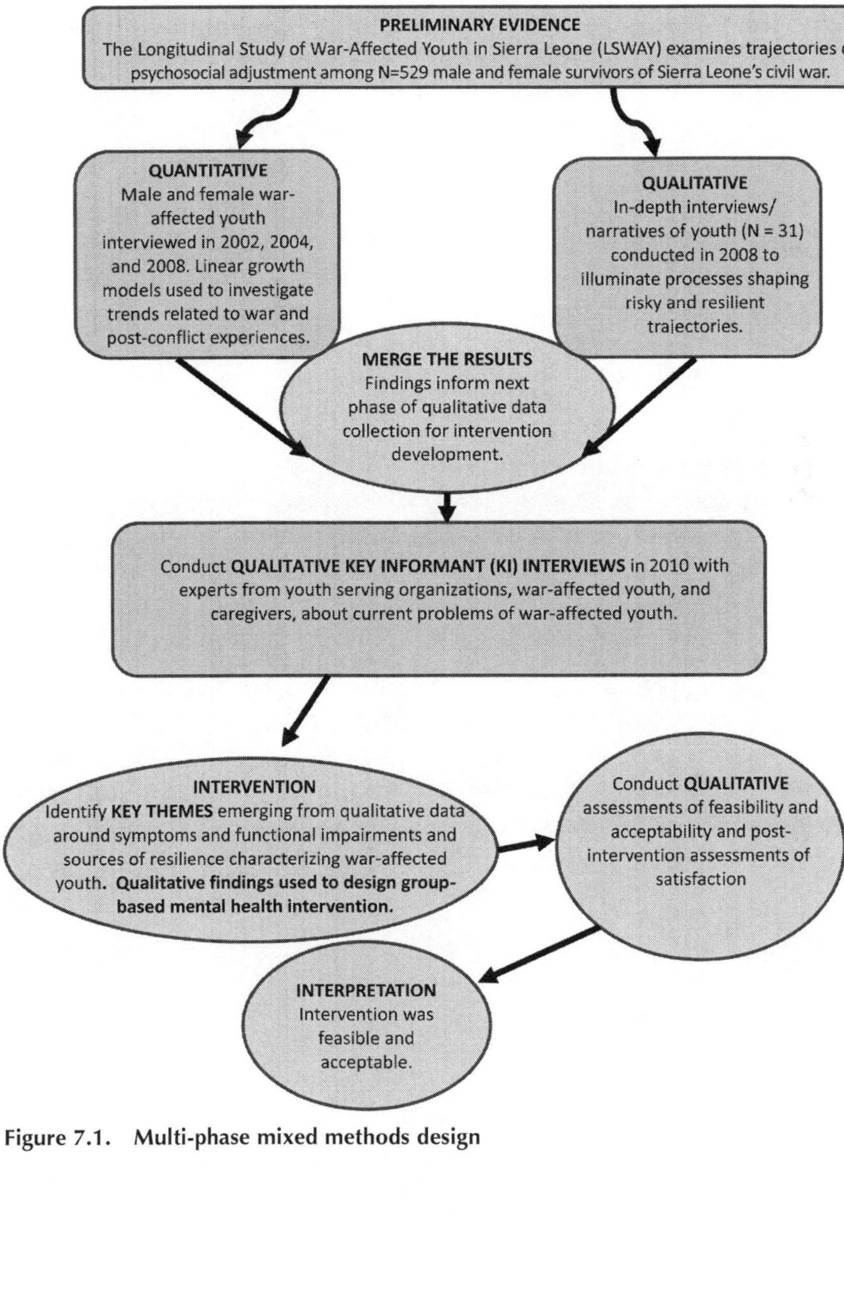

Figure 7.1. Multi-phase mixed methods design

(LSWAY) in the region. Implemented over three waves of assessment from 2002–2008, LSWAY has examined trajectories of psychosocial adjustment among N=529 male and female survivors of Sierra Leone's eleven-year civil war including former child soldiers (male and female) and other war-affected youth. Findings from this ongoing research have documented the consequences of youth involvement in armed groups (often by force) in various capacities (Betancourt et al., under review; Betancourt, Agnew-Blais, Gilman, Williams & Ellis, 2010; Betancourt et al., 2010; Betancourt et al., 2013). On average, former child soldiers in the sample were abducted as children and held captive for more than two years (Betancourt, Borisova et al., 2010; Betancourt, Brennan, Rubin-Smith, Fitzmaurice & Gilman, 2010). Our data demonstrate the multiple forms of violence exposure and loss experienced by youth in this setting: both child soldiers and youth affected by war who were not with armed groups reported witnessing raids, killings, and the loss of loved ones. Approximately a quarter of the sample participated in injuring or killing another person; rape was also common, affecting 13.2 percent of the total sample (Betancourt et al., 2013). Nearly a quarter of the sample reported the death of a parent (Betancourt et al., 2013). Youth exposed to extreme violence (Garner et al., 2012; Shonkoff et al., 2012), such as rape and being forced to injure and kill others, were at increased risk for functional impairments as well as internalizing and externalizing problems (Betancourt, Agnew-Blais et al., 2010; Betancourt, Borisova, de la Soudière & Williamson, 2011; Betancourt, Brennan et al., 2010; Betancourt et al., 2013).

However, the mental health of war-affected youth in our cohort was influenced not only by past war experiences but also by post-conflict adversities and resources. Post-conflict risk factors such as experiencing stigma due to being a former child soldier as well as family abuse and neglect contributed to worse outcomes independent of other variables (Betancourt, Agnew-Blais et al., 2010), while protective factors such as staying in school, having adequate social support, and experiencing community acceptance partially mitigated the risk (Betancourt, Agnew-Blais et al., 2010; Betancourt, Borisova et al., 2010). Having access to school and social support were linked to better psychosocial adjustment and prosocial behaviors which are seen as critical to healthy reintegration following adverse experiences (Betancourt, Brennan et al., 2010).

PHASE I: QUALITATIVE RESEARCH TO INFORM INTERVENTION DEVELOPMENT

The research team collected qualitative data to address questions relevant to intervention development, including: What ongoing symptoms and functional impairments pose barriers to life success among war affected youth? What sources of resilience characterize war-affected youth that can serve as strengths to emphasize in intervention development? What modalities of delivery are most salient to this setting? What potential barriers to and facilitators of intervention delivery bear consideration? Each of these domains were explored among both war-affected youth and caregivers as well as professionals working in the field of war-affected youth and mental health. For those working professionally with war-affected youth, we added an additional area of questioning: What intervention components deserve priority attention to best address the needs of war-affected youth in the post-conflict setting?

Qualitative Sample

To address our central research questions we conducted key informant interviews with youth and adult community members. Through connections with local NGO partners a sample of war-affected youth (N=21), balanced by age and gender, as well as a sample of caregivers (N=19), balanced by gender, was identified. Expert participants were eight local and international experts in complex trauma treatment identified through our collaborative networks from the Ministry of Health and non-governmental organizations providing mental health services. Once initial ideas for intervention targets and content were identified, members of a Community Advisory Board (CAB) met three times to review and discuss findings, implications for intervention content, and potential barriers to and facilitators of treatment engagement and retention. Our local CAB included parents, youth, representatives of local family support units in the police, teachers, and staff from youth serving organizations.

Key Informant Interviews

With informed consent one-to-one key informant (KI) interviews were conducted and recorded by trained local research assistants at a location convenient to participants. A semi-structured interview guide was employed to investigate common problems facing war-affected youth in the post-conflict environment, areas of ongoing psychosocial difficulty or functional impairments, as well as intervention elements or modalities seen as important for intervention development. Interviews with experts working on youth issues were held either by phone or face to face. These experts also reviewed a summary sheet laying out the initial intervention components under consideration and commented on their appropriateness to the Sierra Leone context and the target population. Each KI interview took about one to two hours to complete. All interviews were transcribed, translated, and stored on encrypted computers. All study methods were reviewed and obtained research ethics approval from affiliated Institutional Review Boards.

Analysis of the Qualitative Data

Qualitative data analysis was informed by Grounded Theory techniques (Miles & Huberman, 1994; Strauss & Corbin, 1990) and a four-step analytical strategy derived from Content Analysis (Creswell, 2009; Smith, 1992). First, we used open-coding to examine key themes in the data (e.g., current issues relevant to war-affected youth, clinical suitability of treatment components, improving youth access to services). Second, we iteratively developed a coding scheme organized by key themes. Third, two team members trained in the coding scheme independently coded 10 percent of transcripts to examine reliability. Poor agreement was grounds for refining the code book and retraining until coding was at 80 percent agreement. Fourth, team members coded the full dataset in NVivo (QSR International, 2010) using the robust coding scheme. Results provided a deeper understanding of the delivery context and strategies for improving youth engagement and retention. Results also provided data on how to integrate the Youth Readiness Intervention (YRI) into other community services such as education and employment programs and was a cross-check of the clinical relevance and acceptability of the suggested YRI components.

Qualitative Findings

Overall, the qualitative data triangulated our prior quantitative findings, revealing that those war-affected youth who continue to struggle in the post-conflict environment demonstrate a range of comorbid problems: symptoms of depression and hopelessness; traumatic stress reactions manifest as problems with emotion regulation and anger; as well as difficulties in interpersonal relationships. Risky coping behaviors, such as drug and alcohol use, theft, physical fighting, intimate partner violence, and transactional sex were frequently reported. Further, youth and adult KIs often indicated that these behaviors were worsened by negative peer influences, poor social support and poverty. One caregiver stated, "*The drug habit has become notorious now. The use of* diamba *and cannabis is all over the place, as well as prostitution, abusive language, disrespect for elders, and theft*" (male, forty years). Another caregiver reported, "*Their attitude to life is bad. Nobody motivates them. They just seem to be abandoned.*"

These difficulties posed barriers for youth trying to access the few opportunities for education or employment available. For example, when asked whether the youth in her community had any goals in life, one sixteen-year-old female youth participant replied, "*They do, but they do not have the means to realize them.*" An expert reported that youth "*easily drop out [of school], because they still don't . . . have the kind of coping mechanisms they really require to face challenges.*" Our study findings also suggest that malleable protective factors (e.g., social support, determination, coping skills, school involvement, employment, and positive peer relationships) could be leveraged by interventions to improve mental health outcomes among youth.

Qualitative findings indicated that planned interventions should focus on the multitude of severe stressors facing youth in post-conflict environments. For instance, one expert key informant emphasized, "*I think they are more traumatized by the day-to-day frustrations of poverty and lack of perspective than the war traumas.*" In addition, the concept of readiness was mentioned by twenty-seven participants (56.3 percent). One expert informant suggested that "*merely sending them to school still creates some challenges . . . they easily drop out, because they still don't [have] the kind of the coping mechanisms they really require to face challenges.*" Interviews with key informant experts from youth-serving agencies also revealed several contextual realities relevant for intervention design: first, limited human resources mandated delivery in groups by counselors with a very basic level of mental health training (high-school completion minimum, with some training and experience in counseling). Second, comorbidity and histories of complex and repeated trauma would need to inform service development as single disorder-focused interventions might not meet the needs of youth struggling with a variety of comorbid issues and ongoing threats to safety and security. Third, the intervention would need to link to opportunities for employment or education in order to have lasting effects. A summary of themes arising from the qualitative data is available in table 7.1.

PHASE II: APPLICATION OF FINDINGS: DEVELOPING THE YOUTH READINESS INTERVENTION

Building on our quantitative and qualitative findings, the Youth Readiness Intervention (YRI) was developed to embody what Herman (2001) refers to as a "Stage 1" trauma intervention intended to stabilize youth, ensure their safety, build healthy emotion-regulation practices, and strengthen skills for managing painful memories and experiences. In the literature on trauma and recovery Stage 1 treatments target coping skills, immediate symptom alleviation, and healthier day-to-day functioning; they can also serve as prerequisites for intensive Stage 2 trauma-focused

Table 7.1. Themes emerging from qualitative data interviews of youth, caregivers, and experts

Theme	*Youth N (%)*	*Adults N (%)*	*Experts N (%)*	*Illustrative Quotes*
Common Symptoms and Functional Impairments				
Risky behaviors	20 (95.2)	17 (89.5)	8 (100)	"Many things happen in a country after a war experience . . . and what is happening around now is different, such as theft, at the scale and level it is carried out, fighting with weapons, which has also become rampant." Female, thirty-two years, expert informant. "For men, it is the drugs, and prostitution for the girls, as they have ended up being responsible for themselves with no one to care for them." Female, twenty-three years, youth. "It is similar for both boys and girls, and most of the girls have taken to drinking, smoking, and are into every bad way of life, because they have not been able to achieve for themselves." Female, forty-five years, parent.
Bad behaviors/ waywardness	17 (81)	11 (57.9)	5 (62.5)	"On the whole, if you look at the lives of the young boys and girls, it is not good because some are living wayward lives and some lives do not commensurate to the expectation of the community. . . . Some look at their past and indulge into a way of life similar to how it was before and just as wayward." Male, thirty-five years, parent. "Since the end of the war, peer influence has been great on the youths. For those coming from undisciplined homes, the peer influence has made them wayward and even for those who come from disciplined homes, it tends to mold them into what it wants them to be." Female, thirty-nine years, parent. "Some youths ran off with the rebels and copied waywardness and upon their return have been disrespectful of the elders and behave just as they choose." Female, twenty-three years, youth. "The life the children are living today is not pleasing as a parent because the children have lost focus after the war. They are living as they please not consulting parents or doing anything for their own future. They are living life as if life is only about waking up and sleeping, and they do not plan for the future." Male, fifty-two years, parent.

Aggressive behaviors	8 (38.1)	13 (68.4)	7 (87.5)	"Some of those who fought the war tend to want to learn new ways of life, whereas others tend to be living violent lives, reliving their violent past, stealing from people." Female, thirty-two years, expert. "There is poverty, youths are engaged in fighting, which is all we see." Female, forty-two years, parent. "Youths have become more violent and theft has become an order of the day in the lives of the youths and the way of life is breeding suffering in the country." Female, thirty-eight years, parent. "Interestingly, within a [social] group, there is so much tendency for violence because your status within the group is being justified by how violent, how bold, how strong you are, it actually encourages children to be violent." Male, thirty-eight years, expert.
Trauma/ re-experiencing	6 (28.6)	4 (21.1)	5 (62.5)	"Youths who participated in the war are mostly known to re-experience, and relive the experiences of the war." Female, twenty-three, youth. "It is really about getting over the trauma of the war, and there are some youth who have eventually found it difficult to move on to learn something new in their lives." Female, twenty-three, youth.
Bad attitudes	4 (19)	6 (31.6)	4 (50)	"I can say that what they are experiencing is so miserable for now . . . what we see in Kono is that the bad attitude of youths is not encouraging." Male, twenty years, youth. "Some are very disrespectful to their elders." Male, eighteen years, youth. "Their attitude to life is bad. Nobody motivates them. They just seem to be abandoned." Female, forty-three years, parent. "Some who lost their family live on their own in the street. They are living with bad attitudes." Male, forty, expert.
Frustration	9 (42.9)	2 (10.5)	3 (37.5)	"Some do have goals and for others the opportunity does not easily come by, others play with it and fail to put their shoulders to the wheel, but how to achieve that goal becomes another problem in the face of peer influence." Female, thirty-nine years, parent. "Some youths are known to have frostrate (locally derived term for distress) because they could not achieve their future goals, especially when they see their friends with whom they began having climbed up the heights of success." Female, twenty-three years, youth.

(continued)

Table 7.1. *(Continued)*

Theme	*Youth N (%)*	*Adults N (%)*	*Experts N (%)*	*Illustrative Quotes*
Interpersonal problems	5 (23.8)	4 (21.1)	4 (50)	"They may quarrel over one person getting an advantage over the others, like getting a job when the other cannot." Female, seventeen years, youth. "These are groups of children that come together, well, with a perceived aim of socializing . . . but then you have a lot of tension and conflict . . . within the groups themselves." Male, thirty-eight years, expert. "Girls normally have a lot of problems with relationships, even domestic relationships . . . and they are really very sensitive." Male, thirty-eight years, expert. "It has not been easy since the love that existed among certain people turned to feuds between people after the loss of their relatives during the war. That usually manifested when certain conversations came up among them. There has been no love among the youth and in Sierra Leone in general." Male, twenty-five years, expert.
Hopelessness	1 (4.8) --	5 (26.3)	4 (50)	"There has not been hope for the future [among Sierra Leonean youth]." Female, forty-three years, parent. "Some girls would have been raped and come to have a negative attitude toward men, not taking life seriously again." Female, forty-three years, parent. "There are no jobs, and they cannot become somebody in the community, there has been evidence like that of one youth in [a town] who hung himself with a rope as a result of hardship." Female, thirty-three years, parent.
Common Sources of Resilience				
Goal-setting	11 (52.4)	11 (57.9)	7 (87.5)	"Some youths want to be somebody in life and even though they do not have financial support, want training in skills." Female, twenty-three years, youth. "They plan to go to school, to better themselves, to conduct successful business, to make something out of their life." Female, thirty-one years, parent.

Determination	7 (33.3)	13 (68.4)	5 (62.5)	"[The key to success is] determination to be something in life and working toward it." Female, twenty-three years, youth. "Some are trying really and some have known that they need to change from the past life in which they committed evil, and some are doing well in it." Female, forty-five years, parent. "I will advise the school going youths to continue going to school, and those working and going to school to keep at their schooling, as one does not run and scratch his feet at the same time." Female, sixteen years, youth.
Peer support	10 (47.6)	6 (31.6)	7 (87.5)	"You see there is a group of wayward boys living in my area. These boys came out of the war and are not working. They formed themselves into a group, calling themselves good Samaritans. During the road construction in which vehicles use the bypass which is rugged, the group of boys use the bricks from the broken walls to fill the pothole and make the road fine and solicited help from the motorist, which they later shared among themselves to eat. They also organized themselves to go out asking for odds jobs like painting to earn money." Male, fifty-two years, parent "So it's like, in a common slogan, 'fire from the riverside, where do you run for help?' And you find out that these are the reasons why children form their own groups in communities and society, only to get support from one another." Male, thirty-eight years, expert.
Individual resilience/ Succeeding against odds/ Helping oneself	10 (47.6)	9 (47.4)	3 (37.5)	"[In speaking of a resilient youth] He has a very strong sense of: I want to succeed in life, and however these people treat me I have to be grateful because they took me in. So he was always trying to show that gratefulness to them, and he was patient, and he made it, and in the end people are amazed and respectful a lot, because he was able to make it." Female, expert. "The only I thing I think someone can do is to encourage the person to know that all hope is not lost in the face of the situation they are going through." Female, thirty-two years, expert. Key qualities for success among youth include: "He can be ambitious." Female, forty-five years, parent. "He would have a content mind to give him the knowledge." Female, twenty-nine years, parent. "They are courageous." Female, twenty-five years, parent.

interventions (Herman, 2001; Silva et al., 2003). In this manner the YRI builds upon a number of effective CBT components including psychoeducation, behavioral activation, relaxation, cognitive reframing, mood monitoring and interpersonal skills. The STAIR manual developed by Cloitre and colleagues (Cloitre, Koenen, Cohen & Han, 2002) served as an additional model in developing the YRI and its sequencing. Treatment components addressing interpersonal deficits were drawn from group interpersonal therapy (IPT-G) following the first author's experience with delivering this intervention to youth in northern Uganda (Betancourt et al., 2012; Bolton et al., 2007), and the salience of interpersonal difficulties for the lasting effects of war in the lives of youth from our qualitative data.

As a Stage 1 treatment the YRI intervention components reflect three stages common to trauma-focused evidence based treatments: stabilization, integration, and connection (Cloitre, 2008). In the *stabilization* phase common practice elements (e.g., affect identification, emotion regulation, and coping skills) are taught and practiced. In the *integration* phase trauma psychoeducation and narrative discussion of moving from past to future goals and productive problem solving are critical elements. In the *connection* phase interpersonal and communication skills are discussed and practiced in group along with methods for navigating challenges in interpersonal relationships. The final YRI sessions are future-focused and include monitoring and acknowledging progress throughout the intervention. These common treatment elements have demonstrated effectiveness in prior intervention work with multisymptomatic youth (Barlow, Allen & Choate, 2004; Chorpita, Daleiden & Weisz, 2005; Weisz, Hawley & Jensen-Doss, 2004; Wilamowska et al., 2010). Given our consultation with experts in Sierra Leone, popular Krio phrases was used in the session titles to reflect the content and help youth understand each technique (see table 7.2).

To prepare the intervention for use in Sierra Leone, evidence-based techniques drawn from cognitive behavioral therapy, and group interpersonal therapy were adapted specifically for this low-resource setting and context. Modifications were required. For example, given the low literacy levels in the region the common practice of assigning homework for youth engaged in treatment was modified; instead of written material, participants were encouraged to practice skills learned in the group within their peer and family relationships between sessions. The results of practice were then reviewed through discussion and verbal reports. A number of common practice elements were adapted to fit the local context. For instance, deep belly (diaphragmatic) breathing was introduced and practiced as a relaxation skill in group. Participants were instructed to practice it at least once during the intervening week when they encountered a stressful interaction or situation and then returned to group to discuss their experiences using the technique. As another example, a thermometer is often used in more developed countries as a metaphor for monitoring moods. However, in Sierra Leone few youth are familiar with thermometers, making the analogy difficult to transfer. Thus, the group discussed potential metaphors for monitoring emotion. It was determined from our qualitative data that anger (termed *vex* in Krio) was a key emotion that youth struggled with and that a pot of boiling water (reacting to increases and decreases in heat) or a radio (for which the volume can be turned up or down) would be more appropriate guiding metaphors. The clinical team tested these metaphors in group sessions discussing how to watch for triggers for anger and implement relaxation and cognitive restructuring in a preventive fashion. Ultimately the metaphor of boiling water was seen as most effective at communicating the concept and was used in the manual.

Finally, a group treatment was considered the most appropriate delivery mode. Group interventions are useful in settings where few human resources for mental health exist. Group therapy has the potential to normalize difficult experiences and highlight progress through witnessing change in others. Groups can also encourage peer-to-peer learning and social connections that can contribute to sustaining the intervention's impact by providing social support long after treatment ends (Bass et al., 2006).

PHASE III: ASSESSING INTERVENTION FEASIBILITY, ACCEPTABILITY, AND SATISFACTION

To evaluate the feasibility of the YRI an open trial of the intervention was conducted among N=32 youth stratified by age (fifteen to seventeen and eighteen to twenty-four years old) and gender (male and female); four groups in total. Following a strong demonstration of feasibility and initial effectiveness the intervention was tested in a randomized controlled trial conducted in Sierra Leone's capital Freetown (Betancourt et al. Under review). Improvements in outcomes among YRI participants (n=436, ages fifteen to twenty-four years old, 54 percent female) were further supported through analysis of post-intervention qualitative interviews conducted with a randomly selected subsample of youth participants (n=9). Many reported clinically meaningful improvements in emotion regulation and were able to discern the appropriate skills for specific situations; for example one youth participant stated: "*whenever I'm involved in an argument, I get nervous or shocked, I usually . . . [use communication skills] or do some . . . [relaxation skills] to calm my nerves*" (female, fifteen years). Others

Table 7.2. Youth Readiness Intervention session outline (with summary and Krio title)

Stabilization	Community Outreach and Screening
	Introduce intervention to community Provide psychoeducation on the consequences of trauma to local leaders
	Session 1: Introductions and Building Group Cohesion *"Kapu sense no kapu wod" (Making sense of experiences)*
	Introduce intervention format and goals Build motivation for group participation and cohesion among group members Elicit individualized goals for each group member
	Session 2: Trauma Psychoeducation *"Sabi nor get worri" (If you have knowledge, you will no longer be worried)*
	Provide education regarding the impact of trauma/loss on family functioning and relationships, including how trauma contributes to mood dysregulation and anger
	Session 3: Understanding the Link Between Beliefs, Bodies, and Behaviors *"Al kondo day lae in beleh na gron bot yu nor no wus wan in beleh day at" (If you see lizards laying with their bellies on the ground, you won't know which one's belly hurts—You can't know someone's beliefs without them telling you)*
	Discuss how beliefs, bodies, and behaviors are connected Explore healthy and unhealthy coping strategies
	Session 4: Taking Control of Your Life *"Be yu yone watchman/watchooman" (Be your own watchman/watchwoman)*
	Discuss self-care and taking charge of your life Introduce skills for self-regulation/mood regulation, "staying busy and having fun" and "belleh blow"
Integration	**Session 5: Relaxation and Behavioral Activation** *"Yu kin chenje ow yu fil" (You can change how you feel)*
	Reflect on how behaviors can alter mood Learn about how progressive relaxation and guided imagery can combat tension Identify opportunities for behavioral activation and pleasant activity scheduling
	Session 6: Dealing with the Past/ Things Lost and Things Gained *"Nah we yone" (We own it—The past is part of us)*
	Psychoeducation about grief and loss, and growth in the face of trauma and loss
	Session 7: Sequential (step-by-step) Problem Solving and Introduction to Relaxation Techniques *"If yu tek tem kill anch, yu go see in gut" (If you act with patience you will reach your goal)*
	Introduce sequential problem solving via role play Introduce and practice the first relaxation technique: deep belly breathing

Connection	**Session 8: Building Interpersonal Skills** *"If yu was yu han fayn yu go it wit big pipul"* (Present yourself well you will have many opportunities)
Connection	Explore how emotions can impact an interaction Practice interacting with others in a positive and assertive manner Discuss solutions to problems with relationships
Connection	**Session 9: Review of Coping Skills and Problem Solving** *"If yu nor no usai yu komot, yu for no usai yu day go" (If you don't know where you are coming from, you should know where you are going)*
Connection	Review helpful and unhelpful coping Practice applying problem-solving skills
Connection	**Session 10: Addressing Negative Self-Perceptions** *"Gud wod pull gud kola" (If you present yourself positively, you will receive positive reactions)*
Connection	Discuss how negative beliefs affect emotions and behaviors Facilitate identification of unhelpful or negative beliefs including hostile attributions and negative self-perceptions Introduce strategies for positive reframing/counteracting negative self-image & stigma
	Session 11: Review of Skills and Relapse Prevention *"Timap nor day tap yu for dance" (Have courage to tackle your challenges and you will celebrate in the end)*
	Reinforce self-efficacy and important concepts mastered throughout Allow participants to reflect on group experience and how it will help in the future
	Session 12: Celebration and Moving Forward *"Tem for gladi en go befo" (Time to celebrate and move forward)*
	Review the sequential problem-solving approach and application to participant goals Discuss potential future challenges Review warning signs and relapse prevention

discussed the use of cognitive and behavioral techniques to improve mood: "*When I'm troubled, I go to a quiet place and think about the positive . . . I look for something that will distract me . . . If I continue in that [negative thinking] it will affect my entire being*" (female, fifteen years). Similarly, one participant reported increased social support and use of behavioral activation techniques: "*Now if I have a problem I look out for someone that I trust and tell him or her my problem, then she will advise me about what to do. If it is good advice then I will do it, then I will go out and start playing with my friends to get rid of the depression*" (female, fifteen years).

Others spoke of the impact on aggression and high-risk behaviors. One male participant (twenty-one years) stated, "*They told me about if I have a problem, especially finance, you should not go and steal because you want to solve that problem, you should be patient or you meet with elders around and talk to them nicely for help, that's the idea they gave us.*" Another participant said "*I don't know how to interact with people, I was so aggressive with people, but since I went through this session my life has changed*" (female, sixteen years).

Most participants also spoke about the value of the group in building trusting relationships: "*Because most of us came from the same area we moved together, we came home and [practiced what we've learned]*" (male, seventeen years). A sense of achievement was evident throughout the interviews. One participant reported, "*If other youths go through this process . . . If some of them have a hot temper, they can control it, if they have a problem, they can solve it, if they have stress they can find ways of solving that stress*" (male, seventeen years). Consistent with YRI aims participants reported a change in perspective: "*I imagine the future. How I should improve myself and I should not be involved in any wayward life*" (male, seventeen years). Another participant stated "*Since then [the YRI] people started to say that I have changed. People can now send you, and you go there and be quiet and listen when elders are talking*" (female, 15 years).

DISCUSSION

It is evident that war-affected youth in Sierra Leone today experience high levels of psychological distress, comorbidity, and sequelae of complex trauma. Preliminary evidence from our ongoing Longitudinal Study of War-Affected Youth in Sierra Leone indicated a range of post-conflict stressors that impact youths' ability to sustain improvements in psychological symptoms and functioning. Unemployment, violence, and poverty remain persistent problems. These issues were further echoed in the qualitative first phase of the current study. Frequent reports of interpersonal difficulties, lack of opportunities to formulate goals and enact them, and a lack of adaptive coping strategies were evident in the qualitative data and informed the development of an evidence-informed treatment through a multi-phase mixed-methods research design.

Drawing on qualitative and quantitative data an intervention to address ongoing difficulties with emotion regulation, problem solving, and interpersonal functioning was developed. The resulting Youth Readiness Intervention is a future-oriented intervention designed to help war-affected youth build skills essential for navigating a low-resource, post-conflict environment. The brief Stage 1 trauma intervention, focused on stability, integration, and connection, was acceptable to youth and community members. The use of local terminology helped the target population connect to the content. In addition, the YRI is highly feasible in this and other resource-poor settings as it was developed to be delivered by health workers with a very basic level of training as long as excellent supervision structures are put into place (Newnham, Akinsulure-Smith, Hann, Hansen & Betancourt, Under review). Finally, the use of a group for treatment delivery is intended to build social connections and supports that can be sustained long after the formal treatment period. Additional modules are being explored relating to traumatic grief and bereavement for loved ones, life opportunities that were lost, and modules adressing "taking charge" of one's life.

In conclusion, mental health service research can contribute a great deal to the service gap characterizing most war-affected settings. In Sierra Leone, despite the presence of psychosocial and reintegration programs instituted immediately after the war (The Coalition to Stop the Use of Child Soldiers, 2006; UNICEF, 2005; Williamson, 2005), limited efforts have been made to establish sustainable programs to promote robust, long-term mental health services for war-affected youth (Williamson 2006). Today, 76 percent of Sierra Leoneans are under the age of thirty-five (World Bank, 2011a), and most lived through the eleven-year civil war. Furthermore, schemes to advance youth employment and educational opportunities, such as the $20 million Youth Employment Scheme supported by the World Bank (World Bank, 2011b), may be inaccessible to many troubled youth whose persistent symptoms and functional impairments make interactions with peers and supervisors difficult. Similar difficulties in family and community relationships also pose problems for many war-affected youth, particularly those facing stigma due to past involvement with armed groups (Betancourt, Agnew-Blais et al., 2010). The current study highlights the innovative use of a mixed-methods approach for developing and evaluating a group-based psychological intervention to serve these youth.

These findings have a number of research implications. First, this multiphase, mixed methods study laid out a process for identifying locally relevant evidence-based treatment elements and cultural adaptations that can be replicated by other groups interested in developing and implementing evidence-based practices for war-affected youth in resource-constrained settings. Second, process outcomes demonstrate the feasibility of recruiting, retaining, and serving diverse groups of war-affected youth in community settings with interventionists who have very basic levels of training under a robust supervision structure. Third, our examination of fidelity-enhancing, low-cost methods for targeted supervision present important elements of intervention delivery for use by local organizations and future research.

With a strengthened evidence base our research can help to build capacity in Sierra Leone and other war-affected settings to implement, monitor, and evaluate enhanced psychosocial services for troubled youth. Additionally, as such interventions are developed and tested, they can be systematically integrated into ongoing youth employment and educational programs. In Sierra Leone partnerships between local service providers and the Sierra Leone Government, through its Ministries of Health and Ministries of Social Welfare, are laying the foundations for future implementation of the YRI in both rural and urban settings. Such collaborative efforts can go a long way to address the serious gap between the needs of war-affected youth and the services available to help them thrive.

REFERENCES

Barlow, D. H., Allen, L. B. & Choate, M. L. (2004). Toward a unified treatment for emotional disorders. *Behavior Therapy* 35 (2):205–30, doi: 10.1016/s0005-7894(04)80036-4.

Bass, J., Neugebauer, R., Clougherty, K. F., Verdeli, H., Wickramaratne, P., Ndogoni, L., Bolton, P. (2006). Group interpersonal psychotherapy for depression in rural Uganda: 6-month outcomes: Randomised controlled trial. *Br J Psychiatry* 188, 567–73.

Bayer, C. P., Klasen, F. & Adam, H. (2007). Association of trauma and PTSD symptoms with openness to reconciliation and feelings of revenge among former Ugandan and Congolese child soldiers. *Journal of the American Medical Association* 298 (5):555–59.

Betancourt, T. S., Agnew-Blais, J., Gilman, S. E., Williams, D. R. & Ellis, B. H. (2010). Past horrors, present struggles: The role of stigma in the association between war experiences and psychosocial adjustment among former child soldiers in Sierra Leone. *Social Science & Medicine* 70 (1):17–26.

Betancourt, T. S., Borisova, I., de la Soudière, M. & Williamson, J. (2011). Sierra Leone's child soldiers: War exposures and mental health problems by gender. *Journal of Adolescent Health* 49 (1):21–28.

Betancourt, T. S., Borisova, I. I., Brennan, R. B., Williams, T. P., Whitfield, T. H., de la Soudiere, M., Gilman, S. E. (2010). Sierra Leone's former child soldiers: A follow-up study of psychosocial adjustment and community reintegration. *Child Development* 81 (4):1077–95.

Betancourt, T. S., Brennan, R. T., Rubin-Smith, J., Fitzmaurice, G. M. & Gilman, S. E. (2010). Sierra Leone's former child soldiers: A longitudinal study of risk, protective factors, and mental health. *Journal of the American Academy of Child and Adolescent Psychiatry* 49 (6):606–15.

Betancourt, T. S., McBain, R., Newnham, E., Hann, K., Akinsulure-Smith, A., Brennan, R., Hansen, N. (Under review). A behavioral intervention to improve mental health and educational outcomes among war-affected youth in Sierra Leone: A randomized controlled trial.

Betancourt, T. S., McBain, R., Newnham, E. A. & Brennan, R. T. (2013). Trajectories of internalizing problems in war-affected Sierra Leonean youth: Examining conflict and postconflict factors. *Child Development* 84 (2):455–70, doi: 10.1111/j.1467-8624.2012.01861.x.

Betancourt, T. S., Newnham, E. A., Brennan, R. T., Verdeli, H., Borisova, I., Neugebauer, R., Bolton, P. (2012). Moderators of treatment effectiveness for war-affected youth with depression in Northern Uganda. *The Journal of Adolescent Health: Official Publication of the Society for Adolescent Medicine.*

Betancourt, T. S., Newnham, E. A., Hann, K., McBain, R. K., Akinsulure-Smith, A. M., Weisz, J., Hansen, N. (Under review). Open trial of a group mental health intervention for war-affected youth.

Betancourt, T. S., Simmons, S., Borisova, I., Brewer, S. E., Iweala, U. & de la Soudiere, M. (2008). High hopes, grim reality: Reintegration and the education of former child soldiers in Sierra Leone. *Comparative Education Review* 52 (4):565–87.

Bolton, P., Bass, J., Betancourt, T. S., Speelman, L., Onyango, G., Clougherty, K. F., Verdeli, H. (2007). Interventions for depression symptoms among adolescent survivors of war and displacement in northern Uganda: A randomized controlled trial. *JAMA: Journal of the American Medical Association* 298 (5):519–27, doi: 10.1001/jama.298.5.519.

Bryant, R. A. (2006). *Cognitive-Behavioral therapy for Acute Stress Disorder* (2nd ed.). New York: Guilford.

Chorpita, B. F., Daleiden, E. L. & Weisz, J. R. (2005). Identifying and selecting the common elements of evidence based interventions: A distillation and matching model. *Mental Health Services Research* 7 (1):5–20.

Cloitre, M. (2008). *Identifying, addressing, and resolving the adverse impact of trauma on development among adolescents* Paper presented at the Symposium on Complex Trauma in Children and Adolescents: Treatment Needs and Methods, Chicago, IL.

Cloitre, M. (2009). Effective psychotherapies for posttraumatic stress disorder: A review and critique. *Child and Adolescent Psychiatry*, 32–43.

Cloitre, M., Koenen, K., Cohen, L. & Han, H. (2002). Skills training in affective and interpersonal regulation followed by exposure: A phase-based treatment for PTSD related to childhood abuse. *Journal of Consulting and Clinical Psychology* 70, 1067–74.

Creswell, J. W. (2009). *Research Design: Qualitative, Quantitative, and Mixed Methods Approaches* (3rd ed.): SAGE Publications.

Derluyn, I., Broekaert, E., Schuyten, G. & De Temmerman, E. (2004). Post-traumatic stress in former Ugandan child soldiers. *Lancet* 363 (9412):861–63.

Garner, A. S., Shonkoff, J. P., Siegel, B. S., Dobbins, M. I., Earls, M. F., McGuinn, L., Wood, D. L. (2012). Early childhood adversity, toxic stress, and the role of the pediatrician: Translating developmental science into lifelong health. *Pediatrics* 129 (1): e224–e231, doi: 10.1542/peds.2011-2662.

Herman, J. L. (2001). *Trauma and recovery* (Repr. with a new afterword. ed.). London: Pandora.

IASC. (2007). *IASC Guidelines on Mental Health and Psychosocial Support in Emergency Settings* (pp. 99): IASC.

Jacob, K. S., Sharan, P., Mirza, Garrido-Cumbrera, I. M., Seedat, S., Mari, J. J., Saxena, S. (2007). Mental health systems in countries: Where are we now? *Lancet* 370, 1061–77, doi: 10.1016/S0140-6736(07)61241-0.

Johnson, K., Asher, J., Rosborough, S., Raja, A., Panjabi, R., Beadling, C. & Lawry, L. (2008). Association of combatant status and sexual violence with health and mental health outcomes in postconflict Liberia. *JAMA* 300 (6):676–90.

Kohn, R., Saxena, S., Levav, I. & Saraceno, B. (2004). The treatment gap in mental health care. [Article]. *Bulletin of the World Health Organization* 82 (11):858–66.

Lanktree, C., Briere, J., Godbout, N., Hodges, M., Chen, K., Trimm, L., Freed, W. (In press). Treating multi-traumatized, socially marginalized children: Research of a naturalistic treatment outcome study. *Journal of Aggression, Maltreatment & Trauma*.

Miles, M. B. & Huberman, A. M. (1994). *Qualitative data analysis: An expanded sourcebook* (2nd ed.). Thousand Oaks, CA: Sage.

Newnham, E. A., Akinsulure-Smith, A., Hann, K., Hansen, N. & Betancourt, T. S. (Under review). *A collaborative model for building capacity in post-conflict mental healthcare*.

Peltonen, K. & Punamäki, R.-L. (2010). Preventive interventions among children exposed to trauma of armed conflict: A literature review. *Aggressive Behavior* 36 (2):95–116, doi: 10.1002/ab.20334.

QSR International. (2010). NVivo 9. Cambridge, MA.

Shonkoff, J. P., Garner, A. S., Siegel, B. S., Dobbins, M. I., Earls, M. F., McGuinn, L., Wood, D. L. (2012). The lifelong effects of early childhood adversity and toxic stress. *Pediatrics* 129 (1):e232–e246, doi: 10.1542/peds.2011-2663.

Silva, R. R., Cloitre, M., Davis, L., Levitt, J., Gomez, S., Ngai, I. & Brown, E. (2003). Early intervention with traumatized children. *Psychiatric Quarterly* 74 (4):333–47, doi: 10.1023/a:1026035426446.

Smith, C. P. (1992). *Motivation and personality: Handbook of thematic content analysis*. Cambridge [England]; New York, NY, USA: Cambridge University Press.

Strauss, A. & Corbin, J. (1990). *Basics of Qualitative Research: Grounded Theory Procedures and Techniques*. Newbury Park, CA: Sage.

The Coalition to Stop the Use of Child Soldiers. (2006). Child soldiers and disarmament, demobilization, rehabilitation and reintegration in West Africa: A survey of programmatic work on child soldiers in Cote d'Ivoire, Guinea, Liberia and Sierra Leone.

Tol, W. A., Barbui, C., Galappatti, A., Silove, D., Betancourt, T. S., Souza, R., Van Ommeren, M. (2011). Mental health and psychosocial support in humanitarian settings: Linking practice and research. *The Lancet* 378 (9802):1581–91.

UNICEF. (2005). The Disarmament, Demobilization and Reintegration of Children Associated with the Fighting Forces: Lessons Learned in Sierra Leone. In UNICEF (Ed.): UNICEF.

Walker, S. P., Wachs, T. D., Grantham-McGregor, S., Black, M. M., Nelson, C. A., Huffman, S. L., Richter, L. (2011). Inequality in early childhood: Risk and protective factors for early child development. *The Lancet* 378, 1325–38.

Weisz, J. R., Hawley, K. M. & Jensen-Doss, A. (2004). Empirically tested psychotherapies for youth internalizing and externalizing problems and disorders. *Child and Adolescent Psychiatric Clinics of North America* 13 (4):729–815, doi: DOI: 10.1016/j.chc.2004.05.006.

Wilamowska, Z. A., Thompson-Hollands, J., Fairholme, C. P., Ellard, K. K., Farchione, T. J. & Barlow, D. H. (2010). Conceptual background, development, and preliminary data from the unified protocol for transdiagnostic treatment of emotional disorders. *Depression and Anxiety* 27 (10):882–90, doi: 10.1002/da.20735.

Williamson, J. (2005). Reintegration of Child Soldiers in Sierra Leone: January 31–February 9 2005. *Displaced Children and Orphans Fund* US Agency for International Development.

Williamson, J. (2006). The disarmament, demobilization and reintegration of child soldiers: Social and psychological transformation in Sierra Leone. *Intervention: The International Journal of Mental Health, Psychosocial Work and Counselling in Areas of Armed Conflict* 4 (3):185–205.

World Bank. (2011a). Education in Sierra Leone: Present challenges, future opportunities *Africa Human Development Series*. Washington, DC: The World Bank.

World Bank. (2011b). Youth Employment Support (P121052). Freetown: World Bank & Government of Sierra Leone.

8

Present Status of ASD from Childhood to Adulthood and an Intervention Initiative for Adults with ASD in Japan

Hideki Yokoi, Soo-Yung Kim, Miki Igarashi, Yoko Komine, and Nobumasa Kato

INTRODUCTION

Present Status of Autism Spectrum Disorder in Japan

In Japan, since the Services and Supports for Persons with Disabilities Act was passed, media reports about developmental disorders have increased, and the term "developmental disorders" is rapidly being acknowledged. The support available for people with developmental disorders is broadening in various areas. Based on an epidemiological study carried out in 2012 by the Ministry of Education, Culture and Sports which asked 53,882 children aged seven to fifteen years in regular classes to respond to the Japanese version of The High-Functioning Autism Spectrum Screening Questionnaire (ASSQ, Ehlers et al., 1999), the prevalence rate of children and adolescents who have autism spectrum disorder (ASD) was estimated to be 1.1 percent. This is similar to the rate of 1.13 percent reported by the Center for Disease Control and Prevention (CDC, 2012), and the percentage of students who have academic or behavioral difficulties was estimated to be 6.5 percent.

As in other countries the importance of helping children with developmental disorders as early as possible is being recognized in Japan. The Services and Supports for Persons with Disabilities Act (2004) clearly states that it is a national responsibility to support people with developmental disorders. We have national health checkups for infants and toddlers at one, three, six, ten, eighteen, thirty-six (or forty-two) months with a high participation rate, providing the perfect opportunity to screen children for developmental disorders. Many kindergarten children in need of support are picked up at the itinerant consultation (i.e., staff from educational or welfare institutions visit kindergartens and nurseries and consult on children's developmental and behavioral problems with the teachers) and referred to supporting organizations. Since 2007, the special education system ruled that, in addition to children who are attending special schools (elementary and lower secondary departments) for the blind or deaf, or those with intellectual and/or physical disability, that children in regular classrooms who use the resource room, attend special classes, who have ADHD, learning disability, or high-functioning autism should also be provided with customized educational programs.

Developing systems for early detection and intervention is under way but compared to countries like the United States where, under IDEA (Individuals with Disabilities Education Acts), people can receive service free of charge from birth, or Finland where there is a special needs nurse with expertise in special education who supports a wide range of disabled children, Japan is still in its infancy. Consistent support and cooperation is required from education, health, welfare, and employment organizations to meet the needs of people with ASD at all stages of life.

Before developmental disorders were routinely recognized in childhood and adolescence, those who had been missed during the health checkups often ended up as adults visiting psychiatric outpatient clinics because of the problems caused by their underlying disorders. Many of those visiting psychiatric clinics for the first time and diagnosed as having a developmental disörder are "high-functioning" (have normative levels of intelligence). However, the harsh experiences to which they have hitherto been exposed often causes low self-esteem and self-perception leading to secondary depression or anxiety. That the degree of impairment in cognitive ability is moderate does not mean that they need less support. Rather, lack of appropriate support might lead to social withdrawal, joblessness, or ignorance about the available support and resources to help them maintain employment.

Developmental disorders have been regarded as disorders of childhood and have mainly been dealt with by child psychiatrists. Methods for diagnosing, intervention with, or supporting adult patients are not yet established. Studies investigating the etiology of developmental disorders are ongoing, but support and cognitive intervention is needed immediately, irrespective of the etiology, to alleviate the distress experienced by adult patients.

In 2008, the Showa University Karasuyama Hospital, Tokyo, launched a new outpatient clinic and day care service specifically for adults with ASD. The day care service differentiated its function from the existing one that is mainly for patients with schizophrenia. Since 2008, over 250 adult patients with ASD have registered for the day care service. In this chapter we describe our initiative and findings regarding the treatment and support for adult patients with ASD at Karasuyama Hospital.

Trials at Karasuyama Hospital

As mentioned, Japan's commitment to developmental disorders lags behind other western countries. Developmental disorders came to be recognized by the Japanese general public only during the last decade. With the spread of recognition, consultations to medical institution and administrative agencies are growing rapidly.

Most of the patients who consult Karasuyama Hospital have not been diagnosed until adulthood; only 7.1 percent had been diagnosed before consultation and, of them, only 3.1 percent had been diagnosed before six years old. If a toddler is diagnosed as having a developmental disorder many supporting organizations introduce interventions addressing cognitive and communication skills through programs such as TEACCH (Mesibov et al., 2005) developed at North Carolina University or SST (Liberman et al., 1998) for the acquisition of necessary social skills.

In adults who were not diagnosed in childhood, self-esteem is lowered due to repeated experiences of failure. They don't know how to ask for help and stubbornly resist receiving support due to a lack of self-recognition and acceptance of their disability, often leaving them without a friend or understanding person. For such an adult intervention, techniques for children cannot be directly applied. The difference in symptom characteristics and changes in social adaptation between people with ASD who are diagnosed in early childhood and those not diagnosed until adulthood is a topic for future research.

Although five years have passed since the opening of Developmental Disorders Clinic and Day Care at Karasuyama Hospital, the number of referrals for admission to the clinic shows no decline. On a fixed day every month we can accept a total of fifty new referrals via telephone calls, but every month those referrals are made within just a few hours. The number of patients admitted to the specialty clinic has exceeded 3,000 in the past five years. Of the new patients diagnosed as having ASD, 34.4 percent were referrals from other medical institutions, and the rest were self-referrals made by telephone (see figure 8.1). Not all of the new patients were diagnosed as having developmental disorders; ASD was diagnosed in 32 percent, and ADHD in 8 percent of the new patients (see table 8.1).

There is no child psychiatrist in Karasuyama Hospital, and we do not treat child patients. Diagnosing ASD in adults is difficult (Ritvo et al., 2008). If the caregiver (especially the mother) fails to recall a detailed developmental history of the patient, it becomes difficult to obtain the necessary information to make a diagnosis. Relations between ASD and mood disorders, anxiety disorders, and schizotypal personality disorder has been reported (Kanai et al., 2011a; Kanai et al., 2011b). Diagnosis is made in Karasuyama Hospital by a physician's interview based on the Diagnostic and Statistical Manual of Mental Disorders (DSM-IV-TR American Psychiatric Association, 2000) and International Classification of Diseases (World Health Organization, 1993 ICD-10); an intelligence test using the Wechsler Adult Intelligence Scale (WAIS-III, 1997 Wechsler); an evaluation of autistic characteristics using the Autism spectrum Quotient (AQ, Baron-Cohen, 2001); and the Pervasive Developmental Disorders Autism Society Japan Rating Scale (PARS. Adachi et al., 2008.) which asks about symptoms from infancy to the present. We try to improve the accuracy of diagnosis by also examining sources we ask parents to bring, such as the maternal and child health handbook or report cards, that give informa-

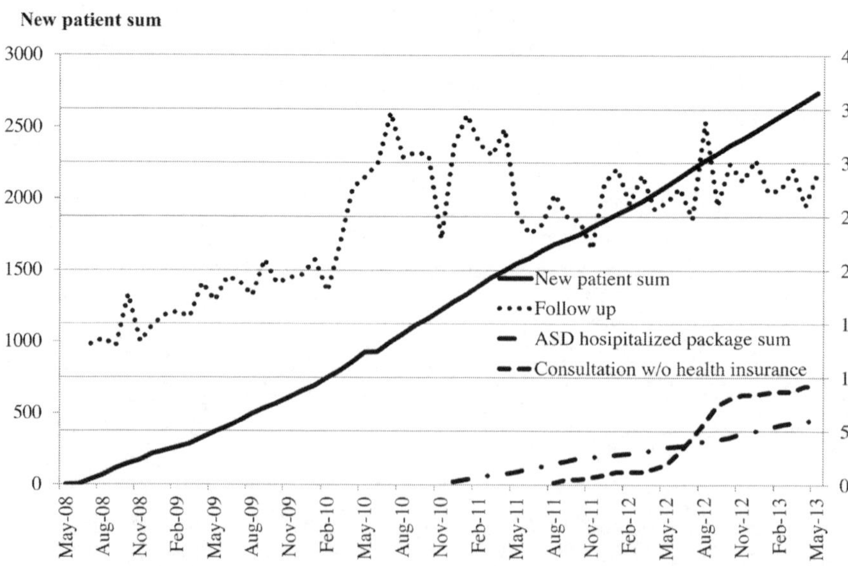

Figure 8.1. Statistics of outpatients at ASD Specific Clinic, Karasuyama Hospital

Table 8.1. Statistics of outpatient (2008.7–2012.6 , n = 1945)

Diagnosis	*N*	*Male*	*Female*	*Age*
Autistic disorder	38	30	8	26.5
High-functioning autistic disorder	96	83	13	25.1
Asperger's syndrome	187	133	54	29.6
Pervasive development disorder, unspecified	296	204	92	28.9
Attention-deficit hyperactivity disorders	163	94	69	29.9
Intellectual disability	90	61	29	29.4
Personality disorders	175	97	78	32.1
Anxiety disorder	268	153	115	32.1
Schizophrenia	102	67	35	31.6
Mood disorders	137	75	62	34.9
Others	131	85	46	29.4
No diagnosis	262	173	89	34.1
Total	1945	1255	690	31.2

tion about the patient's infancy and childhood up to adolescence, as well as interviewing the parent for a detailed developmental history.

Although there was no established knowledge about how to run a day care service for adults with ASD, we started exploring the possibility of providing support. Our ASD support program is based on modified combinations of conventional techniques from SST, CBT and psycho-educational therapy for schizophrenic patients. We make maximum use of their high level language skills and intellectual ability and the social adaptability accumulated up until adulthood, and make sure that day care becomes an occasion for success via learning and sharing experiences.

SUPPORT PROGRAMS FOR ADULTS WITH ASD

Developmental Disorders Day Care

Day care services in psychiatry aim to restore an individual's previous social living functions and provide group and individual support according to each person's goals and aims. In our medical care system the regular day care service, which is for six hours, and the short care service, which is for three hours, are covered by health insurance. Staff numbers are designated according to health insurance policy; for a large day care service comprising two units (a unit consist of up to fifty patients), there are two doctors, five nurses (including part-time nurses), one clinical psychologist, one occupational therapist, one psychiatric social worker, and one clerk required on site (when we refer to day care at Karasuyama, we include short-care service in this chapter).

Adult patients who are diagnosed as having ASD at the Developmental Disorders Clinic and are considered in need of social and communication skills training are assigned to the ASD specific program at the day care. There are three types of day care at Karasuyama Hospital: Daily Life Support Course, Employment Support Course, and the Developmental Disorders Course. There are several groups in the Developmental Disorders Course: the "Saturday Club" is a short care group that meets on Saturdays for members with ASD who are currently employed and socially well-adjusted such that coming to the hospital on weekdays is difficult. The "Wednesday Club" is also a short care group for those who possess a language expression ability above a certain level and who are trying to gain employment. In the groups, members aim to understand interpersonal communication which requires a certain level of verbal IQ. Therefore the "Thursday club" is a group for those who have difficulty expressing themselves verbally and who rarely go out. Dependent on the patient's verbal and social ability, the Saturday, Wednesday and Thursday clubs aim to maintain or obtain employment, and prevent social withdrawal (see table 8.2).

Support Programs: ASD-Specific Programs

There are various programs within the Developmental Disorders Course, but they all share three common goals:

- Creating a place where one can feel a sense of belonging.
- Promoting self-recognition.
- Acquiring communication skills.

We describe below the programs we use for adults with ASD in the Wednesday, Thursday, and Saturday Clubs.

Table 8.2. Groups at Karasuyama Hospital day care

ASD Groups	*Characteristics of Members and Goals*
Saturday Club	Verbally expressive and socially well adapted. 80% of the members are currently under employment. Verbal IQ > = 90 Communication support/employment continuing support
Wednesday Club	Relatively verbally expressive. Verbal IQ > = 90 Communication support/employment support
Thursday Club	Verbally inexpressive and do not prefer large groups. Communication/daily living skills support

Communication Program and Communication Enhancement Session (CES)

In the Communication Program, members learn skills such as "continuing conversation" and "listening to others speaking." Through using these skills they learn "what others are feeling" and what is "socially appropriate behavior." By learning the rules pertaining to human relationships they can reduce the risk of damaging relationships and learn more acceptable ways of behaving. The main goal of the Communication Program is to acquire a sense of how to maintain human relationships. To teach communication skills, we use our original method based on techniques from Social Stories (Gray, 1994), Communication Enhancement Session (CES, Nakamura et al., 2008), and SST (Lieberman et al., 1998). Social Stories have a sentence structure that is easy to understand for those with developmental disorders, and we use them at the beginning of the program to demonstrate the concept of communication skills. After that we use CES techniques. CES was developed in Japan and uses skills based on SST and Social Stories by presenting a situation and a line of dialogue that requires communication skills to create an answering line. Each member writes down on a piece of card a line they think is appropriate for the given situation, and then they discuss and comment on each person's suggested line. Finally, each card is placed on a vertical number line on a white board scaled from -100 ="BAD" to +100="GOOD." They discuss which dialogue is "GOOD" and which is "BAD." The group searches together for the ideal lines of dialogue while respecting the opinions of each member. Sometimes a line of an antisocial nature gathers support from the members, but staff have to intervene and correct their thinking. Most of the members diagnosed with ASD for the first time in adulthood already know what good communication is from their repeated past failures, so most of the time they evaluate good lines of dialogue appropriately as "GOOD." The aim of using CES is to avoid didactic lecturing and help members reach an understanding starting from their particular way of thinking. For those who are not good at generalizing from experience, it is difficult to act on the basis of knowledge learned in a didactic fashion; it is important to follow a process of understanding in a way that is easy and natural for them.

For the last step of CES, we use SST techniques; we set up a scene and role-play the dialogue the group have evaluated as "GOOD." We always make sure to include role-play in our program, because for members with ASD there is a gap between intellectual understanding and actual behavior. Many adults with ASD report that through role-playing they are able to gain new insights and become able to use them in real life. We help members understand the purpose of acquiring these skills through simple social stories, breaking the skills down into several steps, setting the scene, and role-playing. The chosen scene should not resemble a past experience of failure, because there is a risk of triggering a flashback to unhappy experiences.

Psycho-Education Program

The Psycho-Education Program teaches accurate knowledge and information about developmental disorders and helps in the acquisition of coping skills for various difficult situations. Many people with ASD cope poorly with stressful situations and lack coping strategies. By observing how other members deal with their problems they learn that there are various ways to cope with any difficult situation. Especially when faced with interpersonal problems, people with ASD tend to resort to avoidant behavior. With appropriate support, they learn that even a relationship that seems to be failing can be restored. It is sometimes very difficult for people with ASD to identify or verbally express their emotions and feelings, which is also a characteristic of alexithymia (Berthoz et al., 2005). In a program called "Emotional Control," we teach that what or how others feel toward the same event can differ between people (Attwood, 2004). To understand that not only feelings, but also how we think, can differ between people, we introduce the Theory of Mind Task (Baron-Cohen et al., 1985).

Discussion Program

The Discussion Program features themes such as "things that are difficult in everyday life," "human relationships," "what is lip service?" The members share their problems or ideas in the discussions and that helps to promote self-recognition and empathic behavior. For members who have been isolated and excluded because of their ASD characteristics, the experience of having a discussion with someone like themselves triggers the empathic feelings that they may not have previously experienced before.

Peer Support Program

The Peer Support Program has a simple structure in which members share their problems and think about a solution and help each other. For the members that have difficulty recognizing others' thought and feelings, it is also hard to recognize that they are themselves suffering from a problem. In the program we give examples of the problems past members have discussed in categories such as "communication and daily life," "executive function," and "psychological problems," to facilitate discussion by helping members who are in the state of "I don't know what I am suffering from" recognize that "I have the same problem, too." An experience that somebody else would think hard to solve is a meaningful moment for a person with ASD. The Peer Support Program serves as a self-help group for those who have graduated from specialized programs such as the Saturday Club. A group that increases in cohesiveness can progress to hold regular alumni gatherings thereafter and help each other while renewing old friendships. It is not enough to just leave it to the autonomy of members, and support agencies would need to provide a time and place for such activities to continue taking place.

Self-Planning Program

The Self-Planning Program promotes subjectivity and a sense of responsibility by having the members choose a project, decide what part they will be responsible for, make a plan, and carry it out within the time limit. The theme could be anything they like such as railroads, animated cartoons, video games, a specific field he majors in, or a karaoke party, but staff should be sure to support the member so that they can feel a sense of accomplishment for the theme they have taken up.

Recreation Program

The Recreation Program is popular together with the Self-Planning Program. It offers the opportunity to communicate with others through participating in physical activities such as table tennis or walking, or a themed talking program where one can practice conversations with others by talking about common interests such as railroads, animated cartoons, video games, or developmental disorders, or just by playing karaoke or card games together.

Evaluation of Outcome

Two instruments were used to evaluate the outcomes of these programs: the Japanese version of the Social Functioning Scale (SFS-J) for social functioning (Birchwood et al., 1990; Nemoto et al., 2008), and the Japanese version of the Interpersonal Reactivity Index (IRI-J) for empathic ability (Davis, 1980; Davis, 1983; Aketa, 1999).

In the group who participated in the Karasuyama Hospital Program Package, which is a combination of "Lecture/Practice Program" (Communication Program and Psycho-Education Program) and "Discussion Program" for three months, there was a significant increase in total SFS scores ($p<0.007$). A dominant rise was observed in two SFS sub-scales: "interpersonal ($p<0.015$)" and "Independence-Performance ($p<0.006$)."

"Perspective Taking" which is a cognitive aspect of empathy was significantly elevated ($p<0.015$). The details of this intervention trial have been described elsewhere (Igarashi et al., 2009).

HINTS FOR PROGRAM ADMINISTRATION

The aim of the programs is not to cure the disorder but to reduce, if possible, the distress generated by social communication, and the difficulties in everyday life caused by the disorder. At the day care, we search together how a member can live a life of his own and make use of his characteristics. We explore how he can overcome his daily difficulties and at the same time how he can learn to understand and cooperate with others. We will describe some hints on running a day care for adults with ASD.

Group Activity

When the day care service was established, we thought that since people with ASD are not good at adapting to groups, organizing a day care program based on group work would be difficult. It is true that many members experienced difficulty adapting to a group, but it was because they didn't know how to join a group. But they did wish to have friendships. For those with little experience meeting others with the same diagnosis, the day care provided their first experience of sharing interests and accepting others like themselves. Although people with ASD are characterized as lacking or being short of empathic feelings, through the stimulation of sharing experiences with people with the same disorder they may learn sympathy for others or develop empathy.

Group-work interventions addressing social interaction has been shown to enhance social communication in children and adolescents. (MacKay et al., 2007). One of the reasons we chose group activity was that we thought it would be helpful for adult members to have a place to meet people with the same difficulties or ways of thinking, and sharing the same goals empowers each other. In fact we received comments from members such as "It has been an opportunity to think about the meaning my behavior has for others," or " It has been an experience of seeing myself objectively."

To conduct a group effectively, structuring space and time and visualization become essential. To administer the program smoothly, the assignation of members is important. In a program that aims to promote learning communication skills by intellectual understanding, it is important that differences in verbal ability between members should not be too big. Two points to take into consideration when assigning group membership are a patient's ability or degree of language expression, and social adaptability (adaptability to the group). Prior to assigning a patient to a group, we get them to join the group, as an observer. We examine the way they speak or behave in the group and after the assessment we determine whether or not they fit with the group. On being assigned to a group, verbal IQ (>=90) or AQ score (Baron-Cohen, 2001; Kurita et al., 2005) are referenced as well as sex, age, educational background, and social experiences. Most of the adults with ASD aim to get employment or maintain employment, and it is desirable that their social adaptability can be generalized to promote empathic experience.

Meeting Members with Other Diseases

The number of registered patients for short care or day care stands at over 400; patients with ASD are 240, while 160 have other mental disorders such as schizophrenia or mood disorders. The average number enrolled per day in 2012 was 77.7. The average number of users is far smaller than those enrolled due to some patients with ASD attending day care only once or twice a month. Compared to the average number of day care users in Japan, which is around thirty, our service is one of the largest ones.

We started the ASD group in 2008, and now the enrolled number of patients with ASD exceeds that of other diseases. Of course it was not like that at the beginning. We started by supporting one member with ASD once a week within a day care service mainly consisting of schizophrenic members. If the person with ASD wanted to come on a different day of the week, he had to join an existing schizophrenia group. Because the numbers on the waiting list for day care increased, we limited the length of time for ASD specialized group participation to either six or twelve months, but since few members with ASD gained employment or moved to a local job support organization after completing the ASD specialized group term, they had to join the existing general day care service. Their characteristics were often perceived as "odd," and it often became problematic whenever a member with ASD joined a long-standing general day care group that mainly comprised members with schizophrenia. Compared to the ASD specialized group, the general day care group was large, and patients with ASD experienced greater anxiety. We have gone through a trial-and-error process, trying to establish a group where members with different characteristics could remain in the same space and program. As the number of members with ASD grew, co-existence with the schizophrenic members who were relatively empathic was seen to take place. A caretaking schizophrenic member would help a member with ASD, and co-operation according to each other's expertise came to be seen in the program. For example, in a program where they have to give a presentation on a certain theme, a schizophrenic member was in charge of the interview that requires interpersonal communication skills, and a member with ASD who was good at PC work made documents for the presentation. This cooperation was promoted by participating together in educational programs to understand each other's disease.

OTHER SUPPORT

Employment Support and Individual Support

Group therapy programs, such as communication training, are the main intervention in day care, but individual support for each member is also essential. Those who are employed and relatively socially well-adjusted may need counseling in terms of everyday life or using welfare services, but the important issue that most members face is employment. The individual support actually required by those diagnosed with ASD after becoming an adult is mostly around support to obtain or maintain employment. The issues vary among members from fundamental issues such as "Why do I have to work?" to more practical issues such as "How do I write a resume," or "How do I reach the job center?" and "How do I deal with the interview?" We actively collaborate with other employment support agencies. For an adult, getting employment is just the start. To continue employment is the main issue of concern. Although the legal employment rate is defined (companies larger than a certain size are regulated so that 2 percent of their employees should be disabled people), understanding and supportive systems within companies and among personnel management officers vary considerably with many problems to be solved. Even if it is employment on the premise of having a disability, it is important not only to support the employee but also to check the preparations companies make for receiving employees with developmental disorders and to support colleagues and supervisors by informing them about the strengths and weaknesses of the employee and the characteristics of developmental disorder.

For those unaware of their disorder when they were originally employed, whether or not to disclose the diagnosis in order to facilitate continued employment becomes a point of discussion. Conversely many who have failed to maintain work realize the benefits of working under disclosure of their diagnosis.

Employment support for a person with ASD requires significant involvement because changing behavior is difficult for people with ASD. Furthermore, many such supporters in the community, or the employer, have an inadequate understanding of the characteristics of ASD. The manpower required for a single patient with ASD is far greater than for other diseases. Supporting employment for adults with ASD requires significant collaboration and co-operation between related organizations.

Family Support

Providing support to family members as well as to the person with ASD is indispensable. A person with ASD is greatly influenced by his environment. The family living together, understanding the characteristics of ASD and knowing how to deal with his problems, can greatly reduce stress.

The first step in support is that the family accepts the fact that their adult offspring has a disorder. Many families have low self-esteem because they think their child rearing has prolonged the individual's difficulties, and regret the way they have brought them up and communicated with them. There are families who never imagined that their child had a disorder and are shocked to learn about it. Their way of understanding and accepting the disorder varies, but restoring the family's self-esteem based on correct understanding promotes an understanding of the disorder and better parent-child relationships. Parent training is regarded as an effective way to teach interpersonal relationship skills and is a widely used intervention for families with young children who have ASD in Japan; but it is difficult to directly apply to families of adults with ASD. Compared to children who have close parent-child relationships, some adults don't live with their parents, have a troubled relationship, or may be too proud to accept support from others. The individual variation is so big that manual based interventions are not always effective. Therefore, other than individual support we hold the "gathering of families" three times a year for the families of day care members or candidates. We provide support to families by giving a talk mainly composed of psycho-educational content on understanding and dealing with developmental disorders, holding a round-table conference between families, and inviting them to the results presentation event by the day care members. It is necessary for the family to gain minimum knowledge about how to relate to a person with ASD. It is the role of the family to support the patient's progress gaining skills at the day care's small society. Because the patient is an adult seeking independence, growth through various experiences with day care members will empower the family as well. Providing a place where the family can share their experiences will also empower them.

"The Society for the Family of the Person with Developmental Disorder" was established in June 2011 for the families of the patients at Karasuyama Hospital. Because currently in Japan there is no organization that provides support for families of patients within the medical system, we plan to work with the Family Society to change the national medical insurance legislation system.

Couples Group (A Meeting for Partners)

We have a couples group for the person with developmental disorder and their partner. We select couples that are either in relatively good relationships or are cooperative. By understanding the characteristics of the disorder, we hope to deepen the understanding between the couple. In the couples group, the members and spouses divide into separate groups and have discussions on the same theme. The themes for discussion include "Difficulties in everyday life," "What does your partner mean to you?" "Secrets of making the marriage successful," and "Raising children," and after each group they receive homework to discuss it with the partner for thirty minutes after returning home. Both groups experience meeting people who are in similar circumstances and through sharing those experiences we hope they establish and maintain a good couples relationship.

Women's Group

The male-to-female ratio for ASD is 4:1, and women are reported to show milder characteristics (Tani et al., 2012; Lai et al., 2011). We hold a women's group in the hope of investigating the commonalities between women with ASD as they are characterized as having a systemizing brain (male brain) (Baron-Cohen, 2002). Members are women in their twenties including university students with high intellectual abilities. Many of them are good at writing their fantasies in the form of essays. Support is mainly given through the Peer Support Program.

Student Group

With the surge of the recognition for ASD in Japan, support systems for the childhood period are being established and are spreading to include the high school and college period. Because the number of college students consulting medical institutions is increasing, we have a support group for college and graduate school students. Among those who are not diagnosed until they became adults, many came to recognize their disorder through the distress they felt trying to organize complicated class registration and study, and completing their graduation thesis which requires significant own judgment and decision making. The group aims to share difficulties pertaining to college life and find ways of getting appropriate support. Since we think the earlier self-recognition and acquiring coping skills takes place the easier it becomes to adapt to the world, we hope to provide appropriate support during college life and prepare individual's for the next step-working.

ASD Evaluation for Hospitalization Package

To respond to the large number of referrals for the outpatient clinic, we introduced a two-week ASD evaluation for hospitalization package. Those who fell off the referral list or who live in distant areas are the main users. During hospitalization, the diagnosis is confirmed based on interviews and assessment by a physician or clinical psychologist, and their behavior is observed by the staff at a trial participation in the day care program. On the day of admission, we ask parents to accompany the patient and ask them for a detailed history of of the patient. On the day of discharge, we tell the patient and their parents the results of the assessment and the diagnosis. Although recognition of ASD has spread widely, there is still big regional disparity in Japan such that there are many applications from people in remote areas who wish to use our hospitalization evaluation package. It is quite popular because the two weeks are used not only to make a diagnosis but also as a period for rest or re-establishing a healthy cycle of daily life for the adult with ASD. It is to the patient's merit that observation of his behavior and everyday life skills that cannot be confirmed at the outpatient clinic becomes possible in a short–term hospital stay. Those who are diagnosed as having ASD will be advised to use the day care program if needed and to start learning living skills.

Characteristics of the Karasuyama Hospital ASD-Specific Program

There are very few day care services for adults with developmental disorders in Japan such that some travel more than three hours, or even leave the day before, to participate in the program. One of the benefits of having a large number of users is that we can increase the scale of the service. On weekdays (Wednesday and Thursday) there are eight to fifteen people in ASD-specific programs and fifteen people in the programs with other patients. On Saturday, seventy people come to six groups within the ASD-specific program. The greater the number of people, the greater the chances of meeting someone who is like them, enabling the development of empathic feelings. It also becomes possible to group diverse persons more appropriately according to their different aims. We can set the goals of the group to fundamental issues tailored to the needs of the members; Saturday Club for employment maintenance, Wednesday club for employment support, and Thursday Club for daily life support. Those who are not diagnosed until adulthood already have a certain level of social adaptability, or a potential to adapt, and may wish to have interpersonal relationships. Besides learning lessons in the program they can establish interpersonal relationships through making friends with other members.

OUTCOME

The goal of members at day care is to become independent, including being employed. In Japan under the Handicapped Person's Employment Promotion Law there is a levy and grant system for employing people with disabilities for a certain rate (legal employment rate). Countries that have such law-enforced employment rate systems include Germany and France. In Japan, the legal employment rate of disabled persons was raised from 1.8 percent to 2.0 percent in April 2013. The rate is still low compared to that of Germany, and an increase in job opportunities is awaited. The definition and recognition of disability is made through the acquisition of the disabled persons certificate. There are three kinds of certificates for each disability: physical, intellectual disability, and mental disorder. There is no legal system addressing those who fall into the blind spot of the definition—those who have an intractable disease, developmental disorder, or higher brain dysfunction.

A developmentally disabled person with an intellectual disability is provisionally within the framework of intellectual disability and can use its services. Various services and employment systems already exist for physical disability or intellectual disability, whereas for mental disorder the present service system is inadequate. We can see this explicitly in the outcomes of members at Karasuyama Hospital Day Care. Even though all members have ASD, those who also have an intellectual disability are eligible to use the intellectual disability service system and are provided with various services and have higher rates of employment. If appropriate support was provided, most people with ASD who do not have an intellectual disability could find employment and would be highly responsive to support.

At Karasuyama Hospital Day Care, 67 percent of the highly adaptive group members (Saturday Club members) were able to continue work and 22 percent were employed or went on to vocational training. As for the group aiming to get employment (Wednesday Club), 24 percent were employed or went on to job training, and 53 percent joined the employment support course within day care. Most of the employment support groups aim to find employment for the disabled. But in preparation, self-recognition and social adaptability are required, and rehabilitation for a certain period at the day care is necessary. On the other hand, 41 percent of the members in the group aimed at gaining daily living skills (Thursday Club) are employed or in training (see figure 8.2). This rate exceeds the rate of unemployed members in the high-functioning group. As mentioned, this is due to the fact that those with intellectual disabilities have more resources, employment opportunities and training available within the formal support system.

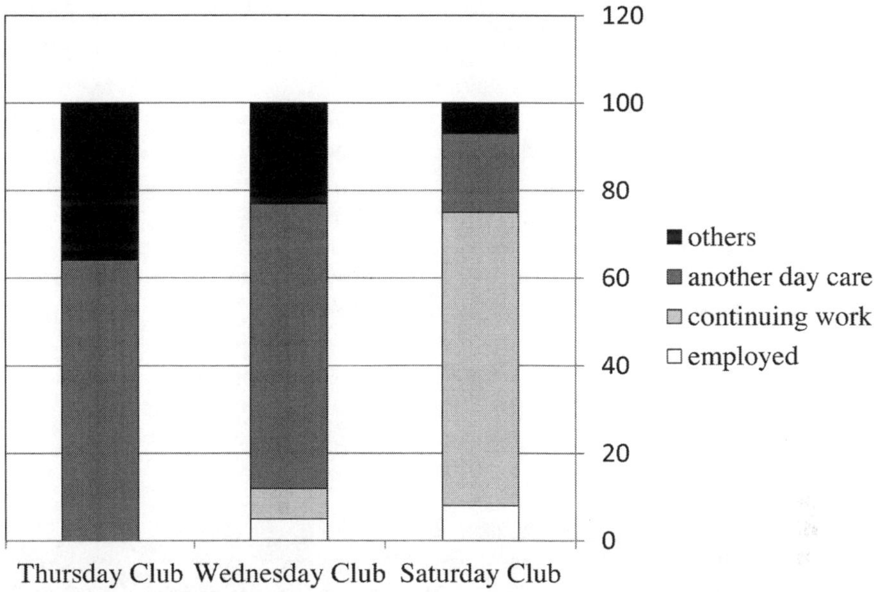

Figure 8.2. Outcomes of day care groups for ASD

We expect to establish a support system for people with mental disorders, too, and increase the number of supporters who have good knowledge about the characteristics of ASD and know how to build strengths.

CASE PRESENTATION

Mr. A was a male in his thirties diagnosed as having unspecified PDD. He had no siblings. He performed poorly in academic and sports areas. He went to college and after graduation has lived shut up in his home. He expressed his long felt difficulty in words such as "I was often at a loss for words," "Words got stuck," "I was hypersensitive to sounds," or "I cannot figure out what other person is asking for." He visited Karasuyama Hospital on the advice of his parents. After a while he started participating in the Saturday Club. At the group he was highly strained and often seemed to be embarrassed whenever staff talked to him. Since childhood he had often experienced his own behavior as making others uncomfortable and angry, and he was uneasy that here too, at the day care, his remarks or actions might anger other members. Passive participation continued for a while, but after his relationship with a schizophrenic member (Mr. B) started to grow, his facial expressions and behaviors gradually showed a change. When Mr. A became able to express himself, with the kind help from Mr. B, the pair gradually joined the big circle involving other members. Mr. A came to enjoy the lunch break without feeling the tension he used to experience. Furthermore, he started to go places with other members after the day care program was over. After participating in the day care for one year he decided to further his rehabilitation by leaving his family and living on his own. After finishing the training course held by the Government Employment Security Agency (called "Hello Work" in Japan), he went job hunting and after a while acquired a position as a disabled person. Day care was the only point of contact with society for Mr. A who had a long history of social withdrawal. By having relationships with other members with the same diagnosis, his self-esteem increased, and he came to understand that what he negatively perceived about his characteristics could be seen as a virtue or strength from a different viewpoint. His self-recognition improved too. As he participated more in day care programs during the weekdays, his personal relationships with other members became stronger, and opportunities for new experiences increased. Those experiences contributed to further increase in self-esteem, and his behavior focused on the future has increased noticeably.

Mr. A stated "I could not do a lot of things since I was little, and I had a feeling of being ashamed about it. I guess my difficulty in looking into people's eyes originates from that period. At occasions when I had to eat in public or stay in a crowded place, I felt nauseous. It was only after a year since joining that I could relax myself at the Saturday Club. The environment where you have an opportunity to listen to the story of someone who has a same diagnosis as yourself and where you will be accepted despite your shortcomings was invaluable for me." Mr. A feels that he has changed as a person, and as an objective index, a rise in his Social Functioning Scale (SFS) score was seen.

SUMMARY

In Japan, the support for adult patients with ASD has just begun. Most adults with ASD have come of age without being diagnosed though they, or others around them, had always felt awkwardness about themselves; they had and are still having a hard time trying to fit into society. Though there are still few medical institutions that can diagnose adult ASD, and though the methods of support are not yet established, a trial of support is beginning throughout Japan. What adult patients with ASD need varies from acquiring communication skills, to employment support and family support. Above all, the role of day care as a place to meet friends who are like them and to share experiences is, for a person hitherto apt to be isolated, quite remarkable.

REFERENCES

Adachi, J., Ichikawa, H., Inoue, M., Uchiyama, T., Kamio, Y., Kurita, H., Sugiyama, T., Tsujii, M., Yukihiro, R. *Pervasive developmental disorders autism society Japan rating scale: PARS.* Tokyo (2008): Spectrum Publishing Company.

Aketa, Y. "On a framework for and measures of empathy: An organizational model of empathy by Davis, and a preliminary study of a multidimensional empathy scale (IRI-J)." *Psychological Report of Sophia University* 23 (1999):19–31 (Japanese).

American Psychiatric Association. *Diagnostic and statistical manual of mental disorders (DSM-IV-TR).* Washington, DC (2000): American Psychiatric Association.

Attwood, T. *Exploring feelings: Cognitive behaviour therapy to manage anxiety.* Future Horizons Inc. 2004.

Baron-Cohen, S. "The autism spectrum quotient (AQ): Evidence from Asperger syndrome/high functioning autism, male and females, scientists and mathematicians." *Journal of Autism Developmental Disorders* 31 (2001):5–17.

Baron-Cohen, S. "The extreme male brain theory of autism." *Trends in Cognitive Science* 6 (2002):248–54

Baron-Cohen, S., Leslie, AM., Frith, U. "Does the autistic child have a 'theory of mind'?" *Cognitive* 21 (1985):37–46

Berthoz, S., Hill, E. "The validity of using self-reports to assess emotion regulation abilities in adults with autism spectrum disorder." *European Psychiatry* 20 (2005):291–98.

Birchwood, M., Smith, J., Cochrane, R., Wetton, S., Copestake, S. "The Social Functioning Scale: the development and validation of a new scale of social adjustment for use in family intervention." *The British Journal of Psychiatry,* 157 (1990):853–59.

CDC. "Prevalence of Autism spectrum disorders— Autism and Developmental Disabilities Monitoring Network, 14 Sites, United States, 2008." *MMWR* 2012; 61(2012): No. SS-3

Davis, M. H. "A multidimensional approach to individual differences in empathy." *JSAS Catalog of Selected Documents in Psychology* 10 (1980):85.

Davis, M. H. "Measuring individual differences in empathy: Evidence for a multidimensional approach." *Journal of Personality and Social Psychology* 44 (1983):113–26.

Ehlers, S. Gillberg, C. Wing, L. "A screening questionnaire for Asperger syndrome and other high-functioning autism spectrum disorders in school age children." *Journal of Autism and Developmental Disorders* 29, 2 (1999):129–41.

Gray, C. *The New Social Story Book.* Future Horizons Inc. (1994).

Igarashi, M., Yokoi, H., Suzuki, C., Ide, T., Obata, H., Fukushima, M., Sano, Y., Kato, N. "Development of the program in the day care for developmental disorders." Research-aid paper of the Meijiyasuda mental health foundation 45(2009):134–41 (Japanese).

Japanese WAIS-III Publication Committee. *Nihonban WAIS-III chinou kensahou* (Japanese Wechsler Adult Intelligence Scale, 3rd ed.) Tokyo (2006): Nihonn Bunka Kagakusha.

Kanai, C., Iwanami, A., Hashimoto, R., Ota, H., Tani, M., Yamada, T., & Kato, N. "Clinical characterization of adults with Asperger's syndrome assessed by self-report questionnaires based on depression, anxiety, and personality." *Rearch in Autism Spectrum Disorders* 5 (2011):1451–58.

Kanai, C., Iwanami, A., Ota, H., Yamasue, H., Matsushima, E., Yokoi, H., Shinohara, K., & Kato, N. "Clinical characteristics of adults with Asperger's Syndrome assessed with self-report questionnaires." *Rearch in Autism Spectrum Disorders* 5 (2011):185–90.

Kurita, H., Koyama, T., Osada, H. "Autism-Spectrum Quotient-Japanese version and its short forms for screening normally intelligent persons with pervasive developmental disorders." *Psychiatry and Clinical Neurosciences* 4 (2005):490–96.

Lai, M. C., Lombardo, M. V., Pasco, G., Ruigrok, A. N., Wheelwright, S. J., Sadek, S. A., Chakrabarti, B., MRC AIMS Consortium., Baron-Cohen, S. "A behavioral comparison of male and female adults with high functioning autism spectrum conditions." *PLoS One* 6 (6) (2011):e20835.

Liberman, R. P., Wallace, C. J., Blackwell, G., et al. "Skills training versus psychosocial occupational therapy for persons with persistent schizophrenia." *American Journal of Psychiatry* 155 (1998):1087–91.

MacKay, T., Knott, F., Dunlop, A. W. "Developing social interaction and understanding in individuals with autism spectrum disorder: A group work intervention." *Journal of Intellectual & Developmental Disability* 32 (4) (2007):279–90.

Mesibov, G. B., Shea, V., Schopler, E. *The TEACCH approach to autism spectrum disorders.* New York: Springer, 2005.

Nakamura. T., Ide. T., Tanaka. Y. "Communication training program for persons with pervasive developmental disorders at Tokyo Metropolitan Mental Health and Welfare Center." *Daycare Jissen Kenkyu* 12 (2) (2008):65–72 (Japanese).

Nemoto, T., Fujii, C., Miura, Y., et al. "Reliability and validation of the Social Functioning Scale Japanese version (SFS-J)." *Japanese bulletin of social psychiatry* 17 (2008):188–95.

Ritvo, R. A., Ritvo, E. R., Guthrie, D., Yuwiler, A., Ritvo, M. J., & Weisbender, L. "A scale to assist the diagnosis of autism and Asperger's disorder in adults (RAADS)." *Journal of Autism and Devolopmental Disorders* 38 (2008):213–23.

Tani, M., Kanai, C., Ota, H., Yamada, T., Watanabe, H., Yokoi, H., Takayama, Y., Ono, T., Hashimoto, R., Kato, N., Iwanami, A. "Mental and behavioral symptoms of persons with Asperger's syndrome: Relationships with social isolation and handicaps." *Research in Autism Spectrum Disorders* 6 (2012):907–12.

Wechsler, D. *WAIS-III Nederlandstalige bewerking, technische handleiding.* Lisse (1997): Swets & Zeitlinger.

World Health Organization. "The ICD-10 classification of mental and behavioural disorders: Diagnostic criteria for research." Geneva (1993): WHO.

9

Why Should Cultural Factors Be Taken into Account in Child and Adolescent Development and Mental Health Care?

Marie-Rose Moro, Jordan Sibeoni, and Rahmethnissah Radjack

INTRODUCTION

Society has to make choices for children, and these are manifested in the medical, social, and political spheres. It is therefore important to specify what children and their parents need, so that this may be reflected in the choices society makes, to help them grow in the most optimal and harmonious way possible. This is more essential whenever children are in a situation in which they might be vulnerable. An example is transcultural circumstances, for example: being born and growing up in a country different from the one in which their parents grew up, sometimes with a change of language and always with different representations of children and their parents, as well as different expectations. Awareness of these processes all over the world has resulted in more and more clinical work been undertaken from a transcultural perspective with respect to the children of migrants and those who, for whatever reason, experience different family structures, languages, or societies: children of mixed marriages, children adopted from a different country than that in which their adopting parents live (Harf and coll., 2013), children brought up far from home, children from traveling communities, etc. Clinical studies of such situations are increasingly being undertaken in many countries in Europe (Moro, 2010), as well as in Canada (Kirmayer et al., 2011) for example.

THE MULTICULTURAL CONTEXT

It is important to study migrant processes, which may lead to changes for the parents that occasionally result in such psychological difficulties that the establishment of parent-infant relationships is compromised. Migration is very frequent in modern societies, which are multicultural. France, where our clinical practice takes place, has experienced different waves of postcolonial migration, and transnational exchanges associated with migration experiences. This kind of movement has occurred in many others countries in Europe and in the world and is now a global phenomenon. In view of this, migration should be a focus of our clinical concerns. Once this variable is taken into account, it becomes even more relevant as the risk can be converted into creative potential, both for the children and their families as well as for caregivers. We try to support this argument from our clinical experience in French infant care, as it has been set up first in the Avicenne Hospital in the Parisian multicultural suburbs and then in the Cochin Hospital in the heart of the capital (Moro et al., 1989; Nathan et al., 1989; Moro, 2000). The ideas and data presented in this article are the result of twenty-five years of clinical experience as psychiatrists, psychologists, and therapists, on the one hand, and of qualitative research (Moro, 2003 and 2010; Rousseau et al., 2011) on the other hand with migrants from Maghreb, Sub-Saharan Africa, and the Sub-Indian continent.

A TRANSCULTURAL AND COSMOPOLITAN SETTING

Our theoretical framework is the ethnopsychoanalytical one, recently also called transcultural (Moro, 2000). Since Devereux (1970), ethnopsychoanalysis is associated with the complementary method, which requires the use of psychoanalysis and anthropology in an integrated fashion to work with patients with different cultural backgrounds. Psychoanalysis contributes to understanding the individual level, and social anthropology contributes to understanding the cultural level of the patient's experiences and account.

This method underlies some changes in the way to assess and provide care as well as the creation of new care models suited in the past for first generation migrants (Nathan, 1986, 1987) and nowadays for their children (Moro, 200, 2002, 2007; Boivin and coll, 2013).These care models have revealed the need for interpreters with first- and second-generation children and families. Arrangements are required for the latter taking in account the children of migrants' language fluency (Rousseau et al., 2012; Boivin, Leanzaet al., 2013). The duration of the consultation and the number of therapists also need to fit with the cultural style of migrant families and patients.

We meet most children and their families individually, with the help of a translator where needed, and in certain cases we need assistance with a group of co-therapists. Although this group pattern is only used in a minority of clinical encounters, it is the system that we shall describe in detail, as it is the most specific to our system. It is also the setting in which we have been able to experiment with new approaches and the aspect that raises most questions because it is the farthest removed from the usual practice of psychotherapy.

When a group of therapists receives the patient and the family, about ten co-therapists are usually involved. In non-Western societies, the individual is understood in constant interaction with the group to which he or she belongs. This explains the importance of the group in therapeutic encounters. In addition, illness and disease are viewed as events that concern not only the sick individual, but also the family and the group. Consequently, ill people are cared for according to group functioning—either by the social group, or by a therapeutic community. The collective treatment of illness or disease facilitates a compromise between collective and family aetiology and individual aetiology.

Health care workers who refer the family generally take part in the consultation, at least the first session, since they possess a "chunk" of the family history. This active presence means the transcultural therapy does not result in another disruption in the long and often chaotic clinical journeys of these families, who in addition often have a previous therapeutic history fraught with difficulties.

In addition to these functions—the culture-sensitive aspect of the exchanges and the therapy, the co-construction of a cultural meaning, and the support for the patient—the group also gives substance to "otherness" (as each therapist is from a different cultural background) and converts this "otherness" into a therapeutic "lever" according to the meaning attached to this by Devereux (1972), which is the basis for psychological exploration. The mixing of men and women, with different perspectives and different ways of doing things, is an implicit part of the system. Moreover, qualitative studies among children of migrants within school (Moro, 2000) or in a clinical population (Moro, 2007) have shown the importance of specific mechanisms regarding children's development that are to be integrated into our theories and practices.

We now analyze some of those results which help our understanding of appropriate interventions in multicultural societies.

WHAT KIND OF REPRESENTATION DO WE HAVE OF CHILDREN IN A TRANSCULTURAL CONTEXT?

With increased migration and its consequences for the transmission of child-rearing practices, studies aimed specifically at infants raised by migrant parents have gradually been carried out (Moro, 2010). All of these studies highlight many things. Studies reveal the importance of tactile and bodily interactions over visual processes which are much more common in the West. There may be a syncretism (or mixture) of practices regarding how the infant is cared for, and the parents may make pragmatic choices with regard to techniques of care available to them—those local to where they live and those from their native country. Parents will look for the effectiveness of any given method above all. Some migrant mothers may have felt helpless when faced with loneliness and doubt (about how to bring up their children properly when they are completely alone). Finally the studies reveal the importance of the parents' cultural knowledge in order to protect their infants and avoid future problems (Moro, 2003). Migrant mothers want to have "co-mothers" at all costs, mothers who will be at their side, helping them look after their child with the support of other potential mothers.

In a context of exile, and facing the unavoidable meeting with other ways of being parents, some doubts may be felt in the ways to parent children, first for mothers, and then for fathers as the children grow up. Generally speaking, the construction of these families is weakened by encountering other family values and structures and sometimes social adversities including cultural discrimination.

Maternal psychiatric disorders have elevated prevalence in the year that follows the birth of children, with an underdiagnosis of maternal depression, as it may be undetected, and post-traumatic disorder. When there is recognition of suffering, there is sometimes misdiagnosis, as psychotic disorders especially are over-diagnosed: cultural and language factors may contribute to these misdiagnoses (Radjack et al., 2012).

We have shown among children of migrants aged from zero to one year old, more depressive disorder than among native-born babies and more problems regarding interaction in the first year. After this period there is an adjustument between the mothers and the babies (Moro, 2000).We have also shown that cultural factors, and the support of traditional parenting roles, were protective factors for the child and his or her parents, which buffered against transcultural risk (Moro, 2000, 2002). This is the first period of vulnerability for children of migrants. The second one takes place at school.

FROM HOME TO SCHOOL: RECONCILING DIFFERENT WORLDS

In the case of school-age children, it is only recently that any major epidemiological study of the children of migrants has been undertaken. Numerical data are often difficult to compare because each research study tends to make use of different categories (ethnic group, nationality of the parents or of the children, inclusion or not of the French overseas departments and territories, etc.). In Europe, the main studies[1] draw very similar conclusions: rate of hospitalization significantly higher for children of migrants than for those of native parents, whatever the reason; more children of migrants are having difficulty with their schoolwork, as indicated in the European Parliament resolution of April 2, 2009, on educating the children of migrants; difficulties in pre-school learning and poor language skills—with the gap widening as the years go by. Poor performance at school is very important, and children of migrant parents have much fewer prospects in later life compared with native children from similar social backgrounds.

Almost 20 percent of secondary-school children from foreign backgrounds are presently in technical high schools trained to have technical skills for a specific job at the end but with no chance to go to university afterward. In a lifetime perspective, almost 50 percent of every generation of foreign children will attend these high schools. In France, some 50 percent of "second-generation" migrant children leave school at sixteen without having learned how to read and write correctly.

To what extent, however, does the disadvantaged social background of migrant families contribute to these difficulties? Many studies have highlighted the relationship between below-average intelligence as measured by tests, poor performance at school, and the low social level of the families concerned. We can therefore postulate that there may be a link between these two factors related to family background: socio-economic disadvantage and the transcultural context. As far as we know at present, these two variables interact with each other, with neither being reducible to the other.

DO CHILDREN GO TO SCHOOL FOR THE LESSONS OR TO SEE THEIR TEACHER?

Social or cultural differences are transformed into their equivalence in the school setting (Charlot, 2000, 26). In the first place, what does going to school mean for a child? Secondly, what does school learning (or doing no work at all in school) mean? Thirdly, learning and understanding, in school or elsewhere—what meaning do they have? Charlot's studies have highlighted one significant difference (op. cit., 26–27): children who are in difficulty say that they listen to their teacher, while those who are doing well say that they listen to the lesson being given. This is how Charlot concludes his paper: "That is something well worth thinking about: do children go to school to listen to the teacher or to listen (also) to the lesson?"

This intriguing question was addressed by the first author, who investigated it in the context of a research study of children of migrants who were doing well in their schoolwork (Moro, 2007). It was surprising to discover that in the sample, fifty children performed extremely well in a school in the north of Paris.[2] With regard to the children of migrants—including those who were doing brilliantly—that result had to be qualified (Moro, 2007). The children were of course interested in their lessons—but also in the person who was teaching them. That initial result shows that children from migrant families are dependent on the emotional aspect of the relationship with the teacher in their school learning; this increases their vulnerability and their sensitivity toward the different aspects of the relationship that their teachers set up with them. This factor may also play a role in the instability of the success rate of some children from migrant backgrounds who, when they move from one class to another or from one teacher to another, suddenly "fall apart," even though until then they were thought of as resistant to difficulty or even as resilient. Many other factors, of course, play a part in such collapses, which may at times resemble fate neuroses or failure neuroses; for example, is it possible to be successful when we identify with a father whose exile has entailed some disqualification in him? But in other cases, there is no psychopathology.

THERE ARE MANY KINDS OF RELATIONSHIP TO KNOWLEDGE

School itself is based on a certain kind of relationship to knowledge, one which is particular to the Western world and which determines the pedagogical methods employed, the relationships set up with pupils and their parents, etc. Like every cultural representation, that relationship to knowledge is implicit yet obvious—every member of a cultural and social group shares it. It is linked to representations of the child, as well as to that of his/her nature, needs, and skills. What should children learn and how are they to do so? Migrant parents, who often have a great deal of respect for academic knowledge and expertise as transmitted by the school system, generally know nothing about that relationship and do not participate in it. Often, their hypothesis is that, in schools in this new country, things are done differently; they suppose that all this is for the best, and they remain at a respectful distance as regards what goes on in school. This often gives school professionals the impression that these parents abdicate all responsibility or have no real interest in what takes place in school, whereas in fact they are expressing a kind of passive benevolence: "this particular sphere does not belong to me, but in my view it is good for my child." Here, too, the relationship to knowledge in which the child must participate in order to learn is that of the school system. This will be possible in a harmonious way and without any superhuman effort on the child's part only if he/she has some help in navigating that particular route—the child cannot foresee what it entails—and if that relationship to knowledge does not invalidate nor disqualify that of his/her parents; otherwise the price to pay will be too high. Some children will not be able to do this. They will remain "on hold," as it were, without being able to accomplish the work of active appropriation that is required in all learning: the gap between affect (family attachments) and cognition (intellectual functioning) is too wide. In order to learn properly, one has to have a sufficient degree of self-esteem and good internal security—and these ingredients depend on one's attachments.

In order to be more specific about the difficulties encountered by children from migrant backgrounds, whatever the causes underlying these, a series of research studies were taken (Moro, 2000, 2002, 2003, 2007, 2012). These highlighted the vagaries of cognitive, intellectual, and affect-related structuring of children in a transcultural situation. In the first study, we have a sample of forty-five children in each group—one of native-born children; the other of children from migrant backgrounds—with no significant difference in their social and economic level. The study showed that, at eight years old, the overall intellectual level of the migrant-family children was lower than that of the native-born children; the migrant group did not succeed as well as the other in some language-skills tests; and they had lower results in a test of non-verbal intelligence with difficulties in reasoning when it came to perceiving shapes, integrating symmetry, and integrating differences and similarities in forms. That study showed that the two groups in the sample developed differently: at eight years old, the children from migrant backgrounds presented more psychopathological disorders, more intellectual and cognitive difficulties, and more problems related to schoolwork than native-born children. Within the group of children who did not present any pathological disorder, there were differences in respect of their intellectual, language-related, and schoolwork assessments. Therefore, in that sample, both affect-related, and intellectual structuring were put in jeopardy by their transcultural situation. Bilingualism is a protective element that promotes learning in the second language (Moro, 1994, 2002, 2007; Baubet, Moro, 2009). Encouraging the transmission of the parents' first language is therefore an important issue for our multicultural European society, as was pointed out in the resolution on children's education mentioned earlier.

These studies highlighted the link between "psychological vulnerability" and the fact of being "a child of migrant parents." However, the exact nature of that link and the mechanism of what may perhaps be a causal relationship still remains to be discovered—not every link implies causality! This research and other clinical studies could help us to consider several mechanisms that might account for both the vulnerability and the protective elements that come into play during the development of children in a transcultural context.

VULNERABILITY IN THE DEVELOPMENT OF CHILDREN

Children from migrant backgrounds are vulnerable; they are part of an "at-risk" group. In the studies mentioned, it would seem that the initial period of vulnerability in these children occurs in the immediate postnatal phase, in which baby and mother have to adapt to each other. The second critical period occurs when the child starts to learn those very important school subjects—reading, writing, and arithmetic—the moment at which the child becomes a member of the society of the host country. The third vulnerable phase is undoubtedly that of adolescence, during which issues involving the dialectic between filiation and affiliation (i.e., the dynamics between family culture and the culture of the host country) that comes to the fore again.

Psychological vulnerability is a concept that was first put forward by the American child psychiatrist, E. J. Anthony, in 1978. There were, however, many predecessors: Margaret Mahler, Anna Freud, and others. "Vulnerability cannot be explained by the child's individual characteristics; it must be understood in more general, impersonal terms. I am now of the opinion that the child's progress along the lines of development towards maturity depends on the interaction of a number of favourable outside influences with favourable innate gifts and a favourable evolution of the internal structures" (A. Freud in *Anthony*, 1982, pp. 13–14). Vulnerability is therefore a dynamic concept; it involves a process that is ongoing. The psychological functioning of a vulnerable child is such that even a very slight variation, internal or external, can bring about major dysfunction and a high level of distress, and put a stop to his/her potential, inhibit it, or allow it to develop only to a minimal extent. In other words, the vulnerable child has "less resistance towards harm and aggression" (Tomkiewicz & Manciaux, 1987). In genetics, the expressiveness of a gene or of a group of genes may be entire, partial or absent; the same is true of this particular aspect of vulnerability. Regarding what will become of these children, their resistance and the interplay of other possible factors must be taken into account.

PRESENTING THE WORLD

In order to understand how this vulnerability comes about, let us take another look at what transpires in the early interactions between a mother and her infant. When she gives birth, the mother is alone in a strange world with all that implies in terms of risk and uncertainty. She will have to adapt to her baby and learn to be a mother without the help of any co-mothers—unlike what usually takes place in traditional societies, in which the group is present during every initiatory phase such as pregnancy and childbirth. In their earliest interactions, the baby will be permeated with the ways of dealing with him/her that the mother brought with her: her language, her ways of being and doing, her relationship to the outside world, her way of taking care of her baby, etc. During that phase, the mother has to deal with contradictory tasks: protect her infant, cathect him/her, love him/her in her own way, and also prepare her baby for coming into contact with the outside world, the logistics of which she herself may well be unsure of. This brings to mind Winnicott's famous ideas about the three kinds of things that the mother or mother-substitute does when taking care of an infant (Moro et al., 1989, 1995): *holding*, in which the mother carries her child, offering him/her a bodily container via her own body, places the infant's body in space while holding him/her all the time; *handling*, in which she takes care of her infant, cuddles him/her, gives him/her tactile, bodily, auditory and visual sensations; *object-presenting*, through which the infant has access to objects that are at first simple, then more and more complex until, finally, the world itself in all of its dimensions is presented via the mother. Winnicott argued that children grow and develop only if they have, from the outset, a mother able to let them discover the world "in small doses" (Winnicott, 1949 [1957]).

Let us analyse a little more deeply the function that we have called "presenting the world" (Moro et al., 1989). A mother deals with the world in terms of categories defined by her own culture. Her experience of the reality of the world is "divided up" and "bounded" by her cultural tools. What she perceives of the world through that interpretative matrix is not a set of objects per se, but the interaction between the way in which her understanding is structured by her culture and external objects. That cultural encoding is handed down from generation to generation. It is on that level, initially in relation to its external aspect, that migration brings about a dramatic challenge: the reference system is no longer the same, nor are the categories employed in it, and all the benchmarks begin to falter (ibid). The impact of all this on the mother is of two kinds: she loses the confidence that she had in the stability of the external setting (the outside world is no longer reliable), and some degree of confusion enters into her way of perceiving the world. She may then pass on to her infant that kaleidoscopic perception of the world, one that may engender anxiety and feelings of insecurity. The infant's reality is built up on the basis of the external envelope constructed by the mother through the early interactions between her and her child. That envelope is made up of a series of operational acts (care-giving techniques), bodily and sensory acts (interactions between mother and infant), language acts (the mother says to her infant: "I perceive you in such-and-such a way . . ."), and psychological acts (the mother's representations of infants, the reflexive representation of the mother when she herself was a child . . .) (ibid).

These elements all play a part in the infant's vulnerability. And then what?

THINKING THE WORLD

In that maternal world, these children will grow up in a relatively well-protected environment. Then the outside world and school come into the picture. Migrant parents sometimes find it difficult to teach their children about the world "in small doses." As a result, every day these children come up against the outside world in a traumatic manner. It is in that kind of context that they grow up and have to move away from their family circle (the inner world) in order to become part of the school milieu (the outside world, that of strangers). This sometimes takes place quite abruptly, if the child is over-protected "inside" and not sufficiently prepared for going "outside." The same situation occurs with children from families who have social difficulties and may be isolated and who are therefore excluded more or less from any way of sharing in group-based meaningful activities and deprived of any possibility of preparation with respect to a world to which they are not particularly well adapted. Starting school—or, more often, when the major subjects to be learned are first encountered, because these represent the real beginning of school life—is therefore potentially traumatic. For slightly different but just as unfortunate reasons, given that children from migrant backgrounds may have to deal with social problems and cultural differences simultaneously, the outside world is experienced as something that excludes. Finding a place for "myself" in the outside world, keeping the one that "I" have inside—these cannot coexist in my representation of things nor in that of my parents. School is the second phase for any necessary preventive measures to come into play, before an early and complete failure in school learning occurs—irreversible and tragic. Through reading and writing, they will come to be part of the logic of the outside world. Some experience that moment as a choice between two worlds, a choice that has to be made, yet it is at the same time impossible. Consequently, they put on hold what they have to say or think—in fact, their whole being. They hide their creative potential behind a facade of inhibition, behavior problems, lack of interest. . . . what a waste! That phase is indeed fundamental, because it determines in an almost irreversible way what sort of place the child will have in the outside world. It is well known, for example, that many children from migrant backgrounds are excluded very early on from the school network, and this puts a tremendous strain on their whole future.

On the cognitive level, Gibello (1988) has suggested another kind of link between the transcultural situation and problems in cognitive development through his idea of "cultural envelopes." These are implicitly conveyed by the relevant culture and shared by all those who belong to a given group. They contribute to the proper functioning of thought processes and to the communicability of the contents of thinking within that group. "Tradition leads members of the same culture to give a double meaning to their perceptions: one that is quite ordinary, and one that is cultural" (op. cit., 86). When we go from one culture to another, the implicit cultural envelopes change, and even if, through time, the new ones manage to be perceived, they are not internalized. In a transcultural situation, implicit elements have to be explicitly learned by the child, they are not given to him/her in the cradle! The child must learn them by him/herself or with the help of a guide. "It is not surprising, then, that transformations in cultural envelopes go hand-in-hand with disturbances in the general functioning of 'symbolization,' as well as in cognitive, school-based, social and cultural learning"[3] (op. cit., 87).

Whatever the difficulties that may be encountered in internalizing that outside world, children—sometimes very early in life—will know more about it than their parents; this places them in a somewhat paradoxical position, one which does not abide with the usual order of generations, and one disrupts it by bringing about an *inversion* of that order (Moro et al., 1989). It is as though these children were self-sufficient. That process is always defensive; it is important, therefore, not to fall into the trap laid by the illusion of their independence. Like other children, they too need their connections to their parents and their emotional links. That inversion, however, is also a source of strength and resilience for these children, as long as they see in it what it really is: a fiction that will accompany them in their mixing of cultures.

THE EXPOSED CHILD

In order to understand the vagaries of this kind of child or "participant" involvement with respect to the external world, Nathan (1986) draws the conclusion that there exists a "cultural structuring," a process that is essential for understanding the genesis of the culture internalized by the child. At the same time, the child acquires both psychological structuring—the "I"—and cultural structuring which, in my view, is not "I am Bambara" but "I am the son of Bambara," an element that implies a certain distance with respect to the cultural structuring of the parents, the distance involved in the mixing of cultures and roles. Each of these structures is dependent upon the other. Although the connection between the psychological and cultural dimensions is set up in childhood, it is kept alive and functional all through life thanks to the homoeostasis resulting from the ongoing interaction between the individual and his/her cultural environment (Moro et al., 1995). Each of these structures implies the existence of the other, and they are all linked together—when one of them is difficult, the other becomes more complex, and vice-versa. Hence the importance of a way of looking at them that is not simply culture-bound but complementary: psychological *and* cultural, with the necessary analysis of the interactions between each of these aspects—the complexity of children's identity in a transcultural situation.

The child from a migrant background who grows up in a transcultural context therefore acquires a cultural organization that is based upon *splitting*, i.e., a separation between two worlds which are by nature different and which may even be in conflict one with the other. That structuring is inevitably unsteady and fragile, because it is not homogenous. In order to develop, the child from a migrant background has gradually to build up the necessary split between the world linked to his/her family culture—the world of emotionality and affect—and the outside world, that of the school for example—the world of rationality and pragmatism. That quasi-obligatory "splitting of the object" in children from migrant backgrounds usually doesn't lead to a "splitting of the ego"; but it is accompanied by processes of denial, to which they are constantly obliged to have recourse. On what objects does that denial focus? Earlier studies have shown that the main object of denial is the family tie and that denial is shared by the family (Moro et al. 1989). The migrants' child is perceived as being a stranger to his own family. At that point, all sorts of fantasies and representations drawn from myths and legends are produced in order to explain the fact of being a stranger/foreigner (Nathan, 1988). If the child does not resemble either his/her father or mother, if he/she appears to have a very good knowledge of that outside world which seems so complex to the parents, their child must therefore be the reincarnation of an ancestor, the gift of some mythical spirit or a divinity of the Earth (ibid) . . . or, perhaps, he/she has been whitened by the White Men, transformed by this society of which I know so little . . . I have suggested the concept of the *exposed child* in order to represent that vulnerability (Moro, 1989). Like the mythological hero who is exposed to some danger to his life—Perseus, Oedipus, Moses—the children of migrants, like those who are adopted from foreign countries, are exposed to the dangers of transculturalism (going from one universe to another). However, if they can overcome this, and if we in our clinical work can help them to build bridges between their worlds, these children, like their mythological counterparts, will come to possess remarkable qualities. That situation will maximize their creative potential, as it is the case of everybody who has overcome some danger, of everybody who comes from a mixed background.

The cultural and psychological structuring of children from mixed backgrounds is therefore based on splitting and on conflict in a context of instability and multiplicity. These mechanisms of splitting and conflict must therefore be seen as determining the vulnerability of children from migrant backgrounds.

THE VULNERABILITY DURING ADOLESCENCE

The third vulnerable phase for children of migrants is that of adolescence (Moro, 2000, 2002). Adolescence is an intense and complex period of identity construction for all the children but even more for children of immigrants as they have to connect, in an original flexible and harmonious way, their inscription in their filiation and their multiple affiliations. Indeed, they belong to the world and groups of their parents as well as the world and groups where they live and it can be geographical, social, ideological, or religious. . . . These adolescents (children of migrants) are doing the subtle work of mixing cultures. Of course, as always in adolescence, this work is not free from clashes, tests, mistakes, excess, transgressions, and risk-taking. They become closer with some of their allegiances; sometimes they caricature them, or they set one against the others. This period made of doubts and explorations is a mandatory step in building their own place in the family group and the lineage, getting themselves ready to make their own sexual choice, and also to choose their alliances in order to establish themselves in a diverse locale.

COMPETENCE, MIXING OF CULTURES, AND CREATIVENESS

The transcultural situation may also lead to unexpected and sometimes spectacular success. That element has hardly ever been explored, although the sociologist Schnapper did so to some extent in her work on the "integration of migrants" in France (1991). In her study of what became of the children of migrants, she had this to say about the "hyper-selective" processes to which they are subjected: "Those who overcome this can benefit even more from it in the logics of self-assertiveness and in the search for distinctiveness—but the risk of failure is statistically high for those who do not have the same individual and social assets" (Schnapper, 1991, 198).

In a sample of children doing well or fairly well at school, Moro was able to highlight three scenarios (Moro, 1998, 2002):

1. The child's background is sufficiently reassuring and offers various kinds of stimulation.
2. In the child's environment, there are adults who act as initiators (guides with respect to the new world).
3. The child has his/her own particular personal capacities and a high degree of self-esteem.

In the first two cases, the initial situation of imbalance linked to migration encounters contextual elements that set up a new order of things, thus facilitating the development of the child's creative potential. In the third scenario, the source lies within the child himself/herself—in such a case, we could say that the child is in a position of quasi-invulnerability, or at least apparently so. Thus, many factors participate in the genesis of vulnerability—the child's own personality, his/her order of birth in the family, parental values, beliefs, and loyalties, etc.

CONCLUSION

When faced with this mixing of cultures, as with any other situation occurring in a child's developmental process, four factors have to be taken into account. The first is *vulnerability* (or invulnerability), representing the child's capacity for passive defence—vulnerability arising with respect to life events and risk factors. The other three elements must not, however, be forgotten: *competence*, representing the infant's (or older child's) capacity for active adaptation to his/her environment; *resilience*, the internal or environmental elements that provide protection (Cyrulnik, 1999); and *creativeness*, the potentiality that some children have for inventing new forms of life, starting from otherness or trauma.

Therefore, to sum up, children from migrant families—children who are truly from a mixing of cultures—are a step ahead of other children, as long as they can discover, in their ongoing development, internal or external elements that will enable them to experience the new creativity that needs to be realised within themselves and with their parents.

NOTES

1. For a review of these, see Moro (2007, 2012).
2. There are a lot of migrants in this place.
3. Translation from French.

REFERENCES

Anthony, E. J., Chiland, C., Koupernik, C. (Eds.) (1978). *Vulnerable children*. New York: Wiley, 1982.

Baubet, T., Moro, M. R. *Psychopathologie transculturelle*. Paris: Masson, 2009.

Boivin I., Leanza, Y., and coll. "Integration of interpreter in mental health interventions with children and adolescents: The need for a framework." *Transcultural Psychiatry* (2013, in press).

Bornstein, M. H. (Ed.) *Handbook of parenting*. Mahwah, NJ: Erlbaum, 2002.

Charlot, B. "Le rapport au savoir en milieu populaire: 'apprendre à l'école' et 'apprendre dans la vie.'" In A. Bentolila (Ed.), *L'école face à la différence*. Entretiens Nathan, Actes X, Paris: Nathan (2000):23–29.

Cyrulnik, B. *Un merveilleux malheur*. Paris: Odile Jacob, 1999.

Devereux, G. "L'image de l'enfant dans deux tribus: Mohave et Sedang." *Revue de neuropsychiatrie infantile et d'hygiène mentale de l'enfant* 4 (1968).

Devereux, G. *Essais d'ethnopsychiatrie générale*. Paris: Gallimard, 1970.

Devereux, G. (1972). *Ethnopsychanalyse complémentariste*. Paris: Flammarion, 1985.

Freud, A. Foreword in E. J. Anthony, C. Chiland, C. Koupernik (Eds.), *Vulnerable children*. New York: Wiley, 1978.

Gibello, B. "Contenants de pensée, contenants culturels. La dimension créative de l'échec scolaire." in A. Yahyaoui (Ed.), *Troubles du langage et de la filiation chez le maghrébin de la deuxième génération*. Grenoble: La Pensée sauvage (1988):140–52.

Harf, A., Radjack, R., Sibeoni, J., Skandrani, S., Moro, M. R. Revah, Levy, A. "First parent-child meetings in international adoptions: A qualitative strudy." *Plos One* (2013) (in press).

Kirmayer, J. L., Fung, K., Rousseau, C., Tat Lo, H., Menzies, P., Guzder, J., Ganesan, S., Andermann, L., McKenzie, K. "Guidelines for training in cultural psychiatry." *The Canadian Journal of Psychiatry* 57 (3) (2011):1–16.

Moro, M. R. *Psychopathologie transculturelle des enfants et des adolescents*. Paris: Dunod, 2000.

Moro, M. R. *Enfants d'ici venus d'ailleurs. Naître et grandir en France*. Paris: La Découverte, 2002.

Moro, M. R. "Parents and infants in changing cultural context: Immigration, trauma and risk." *Infant Mental Health Journal* 24 (2003):240–64.

Moro, M. R. *Aimer ses enfants ici et ailleurs. Histoires transculturelles*. Paris: Odile Jacob, 2007.

Moro, M. R. *Nos enfants demain. Pour une société multiculturelle*. Paris: Odile Jacob, 2010.

Moro, M. R. *Les enfants de l'immigration. Une chance pour l'école*. Paris: Bayard, 2012.

Moro, M. R., Nathan, T. "Le bébé migrateur. Spécificités et psychopathologie des interactions précoces en situation migratoire." In S. Lebovici and F. Weil-Halpern (Eds.), *Psychopathologie du bébé*. Paris: PUF (1989):683–722.

Moro, M. R., Nathan, T. "Psychiatrie transculturelle de l'enfant." In S. Lebovici, R. Diatkine, and M. Soulé (Eds.), *Nouveau Traité de Psychiatrie de l'Enfant et de l'Adolescent* (T. 1). Paris: PUF (1995):423–46 (2nd edition in 1999).

Nathan, T. *La folie des autres. Traité d'ethnopsychiatrie clinique*. Paris: Dunod, 1986.

Nathan, T. "La fonction psychique du trauma." *Nouvelle revue d'ethnopsychiatrie* 1 (1987):8–12.

Radjack, R., Baubet, T., El Hage, W., Taieb, O., Moro, M. R. "Peut-on objectiver et éviter les erreurs diagnostiques en situation transculturelle?" *Annales médico-psychologiques* 170 (2012):591–95.

Rousseau, C., Measheam, T., Moro, M. R. "Working with interpreters in child mental health." *Child Adolescent Health* 16 (2011):55–59.

Schnapper, D. *La France de l'intégration. Sociologie de la nation en 1990*. Paris: PUF, 1991.

Skandrani, S. M., Taieb, O., Moro, M. R. "Transnational practices, intergenerational relations and identity construction in a migratory context: The case of young women of Maghrebine origin in France." *Culture & Psychology* 18 (2012):76–98.

Tamminen, T. "How does culture promote the early development of identity?" *Infant Mental Health Journal* 27 (2006):603–605.

Tomkiewicz, S., Manciaux, M. "La vulnérabilité." In M. Manciaux, S. Lebovici, O. Jeanneret, E. A. Sand, and S. Tomkiewicz (Eds.), *L'enfant et sa santé. Aspects épidémiologiques, biologiques, psychologiques et sociaux*. Paris: Doin (1987):737–42.

Winnicott, D. W. (1949). "The world in small doses." *The Child and the Family*. London: Tavistock (1957):53–58.

10

Digital Horizons

Using Information Technology-Based Interventions in Preventing and Managing Mental Health Disorders in Childhood and Adolescence

James Woollard and Tami Kramer

INTRODUCTION

Technological advances in everyday life, including health care, are evolving rapidly. Many organizations are dedicated to exploring this emerging field. The aim of this chapter is to review the evidence base for the effectiveness of current technological applications in the prevention and treatment of child and adolescent mental disorders.

The evidence for the use and effectiveness of technology will be reviewed across broad groups of disorders: emotional disorders; somatic disorders; autistic spectrum disorders; neuropsychiatric disorders; and psychotic disorders. Where there is no current evidence for use with children and adolescents, significant developments in technology-based programs used with adults will be briefly reviewed. In summarizing the findings across disorders, common features of acceptable and effective interventions will be reviewed. The potential barriers to using technology-based interventions for child and adolescent mental health problems will be explored. Finally, we will explore the potential for technology to change child and adolescent mental health service provision.

OVERVIEW OF TECHNOLOGY

Each type of technology requires a combination of physical requirements—the hardware and software.

Computer-based programs are limited to use on particular computers and do not necessarily require an internet connection but limit use to particular users. A CD-ROM may be required. Computer games and programs for games consoles are included in this category. The distinct feature of this technology is that it is non-mobile as it requires a relatively fixed physical location for the technology and power supply.

Internet or web-based programs require the user to have an internet-enabled device. They include websites, online chat resources, and instant messaging software. They have the potential to be used by large numbers of individuals simultaneously with or without the knowledge of other users. An individual does not necessarily need access to the same, fixed device in order to use web-based programs. The physical location and availability depends on resources to connect to the internet and can be mobile.

Basic mobile phone technology includes mobile phone calls and SMS messages (short messaging services), otherwise known as text messaging or texting, which are usually limited in length. These basic functions are ubiquitous to mobile phones and therefore highly accessible for many potential users.

Mobile applications or "apps" are programs that are downloaded via the internet onto a mobile device such as a smartphone or a tablet computer. They may require an internet connection to function or be capable of running without a connection i.e., off-line. They may provide a link, via a personal account, to other devices running the same program so that information put into a program on one device can be viewed on other devices, which may be remote.

Social media refers to internet-based applications that allow user-generated content to be created, edited, and shared with others (e.g., Facebook and Twitter). This can be contrasted with more traditional media, such as books, which are written by an individual or small group of individuals and disseminated without the potential for direct interaction with the authors or spontaneous post-production editing. Social media represents one of the most widely used digital technologies, including access to information and resources for health care delivery (Lefebvre and Bornkessel, 2013).

Virtual reality (VR) refers to the creation of a computer-simulated reality that may contain some representations of materials, places, or people present in physical reality but can also contain elements that have been imagined. Virtual realities can be experienced through flat visual depictions on computer screens or through immersive audio and stereoscopic visual equipment worn over the eyes and ears. Integrated touch sensation input is being developed. The virtual reality could comprise information received from remote sensors (e.g., video cameras), which is used to create an immersive representation of a distant physical reality allowing participants to respond to it, perhaps through manipulating a remote device. An example of such technology is used in flying unmanned drone aircraft. Within virtual reality an *avatar* is a virtual representation of a person, which may not necessarily represent a physical likeness of a person, nor will it necessarily represent all of their personality characteristics.

Telemedicine denotes the provision of a clinical service via the means of telecommunication technology. *Tele-psychiatry* refers to telemedicine related to psychiatric services. *Videotelephony or video calling* refers to two people, or groups of people, communicating via a technology link that transmits both images and sounds between them over distance (e.g., Skype). A review of the practice of tele-psychiatry in child and adolescent mental health describes a model for practice and outlines the needs for standards (Hakak and Szeftel, 2008).

METHODOLOGY

CINAHL, Embase, MEDLINE, and PsycINFO were searched, with separate searches for each disorder by varying the disorder specific key words (general search terms used for every search—child, adolescent, treatment, intervention, computer, technology, internet, mobile phone, and virtual reality). Boolean operators were also used to combine terms to increase the relevance of results. Searches were limited to publications in English. Where no papers were identified specific to child and adolescent, searches were repeated without those search terms. Search results were reviewed and non-relevant papers excluded—i.e., those not describing mental health prevention or treatment. Further papers were identified by hand, searching reference lists in papers. Additional supporting references were identified using Google and social media.

TECHNOLOGICAL APPROACHES TO SPECIFIC DISORDERS

Emotional Disorders

Depressive Disorders

The use of technology-based interventions for depression and anxiety comprises the largest body of published research relating to children and adolescents. It explores the use of a variety of technologies: computer-based; internet-based; computer-game-based; mobile phone messaging; mobile phone applications; and tele-practice. The research includes case reports, small feasibility trials, and randomized controlled trials (RCTs). The published research is summarized in table 10.1.

Two uncontrolled studies and five RCTs provide emerging evidence for the use of computerized CBT-based packages for depression. They include studies with sample sizes ranging from 24 to 244 participants, ages eight to twenty-five years; include a wide range of problem severity (i.e., from universal interventions for non-referred to targeted interventions for sub-threshold, high-risk, and diagnosed individuals); number and length of sessions also varied. All report clinical improvement and improvement in diagnostic status although levels of attrition are high. There are a few follow-up studies, and differential responses according to developmental and ethnic status still require exploration. Two studies explored depressive symptom monitoring using text messaging, and one delivered CBT via video-conference with positive outcomes.

Further to the studies in table 10.1, Matthews and Doherty (2011) described developing a small exploratory clinical trial of a *mobile phone application,* "Mobile Mood Diary," involving nine adolescent participants. They demonstrated good rates of engagement and positive feedback from young people in contrast to less positive professional views possibly suggesting that therapists have less confidence in technological approaches. In addition to SPARX (Merry et al., 2012), another example of a computer game design is "Reach Out Central" (Shandley et al., 2010), a preventative CBT-principle-based program designed for sixteen- to twenty-five-year-olds to improve their coping skills and resilience through interactions in a virtual world.

Anxiety Disorders

There is overlap between the programs developed for depression and anxiety as some packages were tested in young people with both disorders. Specifically for anxiety disorders, technology use has been limited to computerized or internet-based interventions. Table 10.2 describes the

RCTs of the packages that have been developed for use with children and adolescents.

Five RCTs of computerized CBT for anxiety using four different packages have been published. They address a wide range of anxiety disorders including social phobia, social anxiety, separation anxiety, generalized anxiety, specific phobias, and obsessive compulsive disorders. Programs vary in terms of session numbers, duration, and professional and parent involvement. All studies document clinical improvement although attrition rates were high.

Post-Traumatic Stress Disorder

There is currently little published research on the use of technology for the treatment of post-traumatic stress disorder (PTSD) in children and adolescents. The capabilities of virtual reality (VR) on theoretical grounds may be promising and has been used to conduct exposure therapy in a variety of virtual worlds (Rizzo et al., 2013; Walshe et al., 2003). A small preliminary trial of a therapist-assisted, internet-based CBT intervention for PTSD called "PTSD online" reported a clinically significant reduction in PTSD severity and symptomatology in sixteen adult participants with good therapeutic alliance and moderate tolerance of the content (Klein et al., 2009).

Obsessive Compulsive Disorder (OCD)

The current literature for the use of technology-based interventions in obsessive compulsive disorder (OCD) consists mainly of studies in adult populations using computerized, telephonic, or video conferencing/web-cam delivered CBT, and virtual reality. A review of these technology-based interventions for adults with OCD concluded that results were promising but also highlighted significant methodological flaws (Lovell and Bee, 2011). However, a subsequent RCT of internet-based cognitive behavioral therapy (ICBT) versus non-directive supportive therapy (Andersson et al., 2011) demonstrated significant results with 60 percent of participants in the ICBT group showing clinically significant improvement compared to 6 percent of the control group.

Two studies have looked at interventions in children and young people (telephone and web-cam based CBT). In an open pilot study with ten young people with OCD which offered sixteen telephone CBT sessions all participants showed improvements and high rates of satisfaction from participating families (Turner, C., Heyman, I., Futh, A., & Lovell, 2009). A pilot study of web-camera-delivered CBT for children and adolescents

Table 10.1. Technology-based interventions in depression

Technology	*Study*	*Intervention*	*Sample*	*Design*	*Main Findings*
Computerized Cognitive Behavioral Therapy:	(Abeles et al. 2009)	"Stressbusters" eigth Sessions thirty to forty-five min each	Age twelve to sixteen Clinic sample Primary diagnosis depression n=23	Pre-Post comparison	16/23 completed all sessions 78% of completers diagnosis free 93% of completers diagnosis free at three months
	(Gerrits et al. 2007)	"Master Your Mood Online" Online group hosted by professional eight sessions ninety min each	Age sixteen to twenty-five Universal Community Subclinical or mild depression n=189	Pre-Post comparison	Significant reduction in depression High levels of satisfaction 79.3% would recommend to others Anonymity appreciated
	(O'Kearney et al. 2006)	"Mood Gym" Delivered in school class, supervised by teacher five sessions thirty to sixty min each	Age fifteen to sixteen Universal—whole school year All male n=78	RCT	No significant difference in depression compared to control Effect on depression, attributional style, and self-esteem in those completing at least three sessions
	(O'Kearney et al. 2009)		Age fifteen to sixteen Universal—whole school year. All female n=157	RCT	Reduction in depressive symptoms over time Significant reduction in depression in cCBT group compared to control at six-month follow-up
	(van der Zanden et al. 2012)	"Master Your Mood Online" (MYM) Online group six sessions ninety min each	Age sixteen to twenty-five General population n=244	RCT Waitlist control	20% of MYM group completed all modules MYM group significantly greater improvement in depressive symptoms, anxiety and mastery at three months

	(Van Voorhees et al. 2008)	CATCH-IT CBT and interpersonal therapy fourteen modules	Age fourteen to twenty-one Primary care sample Persistent subthreshold depression n=84	RCT two conditions: Brief advice + cCBT (BA) Motivational Interviewing + cCBT (MI)	MI group completed 61% of modules BA Group completed 67% of modules Reduction in depressed mood ratings in both groups Generalized anxiety reduced in BA not MI Decreased negative affect in BA, Increased Positive Affect in MI
	(Van Voorhees et al. 2009)			twelve-week outcome for 2008 paper	Significant reduction in depression at twelve weeks. MI groups – reduction in thoughts about self-harm and hopelessness
Computer-game-based:	(Merry et al. 2012)	"SPARX" (Smart, Positive, Active, Realistic X-Factor) CBT based seven modules CD-ROM	Age twelve to nineteen Primary care/School counselling sample Clinically significant depression n=187	RCT	60% completed all modules (of those who responded to the questionnaire) Clinical significant reductions in depression, anxiety and hoplessness were seen equally in both groups. SPARX group—significantly high rate of remission (by CDS-R)
Text message: via mobile phones	(Kauer et al. 2012)	"Mobiletype" Program four times daily monitoring of mood, stress and activity by SMS to promote improving Emotional Self Awareness (ESA)	Age fourteen to twenty-four Primary care sample n=118	RCT	Intervention group showed greater increase in ESA and was associated with greater decrease in depressive symptoms. Significant indirect decrease of depressive symptoms via change in ESA from the intervention, but no direct effect
	(Mundt et al. 2011)	Quick Inventory of Depression Inventory Delivered by Automated SMS for symptom monitoring	Age eight to seventeen Clinical population Major depressive disorder n=28	Single-group Parent and clinician ratings compared with patient rating via paper and SMS	80% of SMS assessments were completed SMS results correlated well with paper results in adolescents Author suggest systems should require brief response from adolescents to reduce burden
Video-Telephony	(Nelson, Barnard, and Cain 2003)	Video-conferencing delivered CBT with child and parent	Age eight to fourteen Diagnosis depression n=28	RCT Video Conferencing (VC) vs Face to Face (F2F)	High rates of satisfaction with the tele-medicine approach Both conditions showed significant reduction in depressive symptoms. With the VC showing greater rate of decline than F2F on CDI

Source: Adapted from Richardson et al., 2010.

Table 10.2. Randomized control trials of computerized cognitive behavioral interventions in anxiety disorders

Study	*Intervention*	*Sample*	*Design*	*Main Findings*
(Calear et al. 2009)	"MoodGym" Prevention program Delivered in schools Assistance of teacher five modules	Age twelve to seventeen School population (thirty schools) Universal prevention n = 1477	Cluster RCT	1/3 of all students completed all five modules Significant reduction in anxiety symptoms compared with control group at post intervention and six months
(March, Spence, and Donovan 2009)	BRAVE Online ten sessions for child six sessions for parent sixty min each Therapist contact via Email	Age seven to twelve Referred sample Primary diagnosis of Anxiety Disorder n = 73	RCT	33.3% of children and 60% of parents completed all eight sessions Post-treatment 30% free from primary diagnosis 75% free from primary diagnosis at six months
(Spence et al. 2006)	BRAVE Online five sessions for child three Sessions for parent three month booster 6sixty min each	Age seven to fourteen Referred sample Primary diagnosis of Anxiety Disorder n = 72	RCT	56% no longer met criteria for primary anxiety disorder—73.9% at twelve-month follow-up Compared with WLC, Online and Clinic intervention groups showed significant reduction in anxiety by diagnosis, clinician severity rating and parent rating, but there were no differences between intervention groups.

(Spence et al. 2011)	BRAVE Online ten sessions for Child five sessions for parent sixty min each Booster sessions Therapist contact via email	Age twelve to eighteen Community/referred sample Primary diagnosis of anxiety disorder n = 115	RCT	57% of Clinic group completed all sessions 39% of Online group completed all sessions Online group and Clinic group showed similar reduction in diagnosable anxiety disorder at twelve-week, six-month, and twelve-month follow-up—significantly different to WLC
(Stallard et al. 2011)	"Think Feel Do" six sessions thirty to fourty-five minutes Requires facilitator CD-ROM	Age eleven to seventeen Outpatient clinic sample Anxiety and depression (more anxiety than depression) n=20	RCT	cCBT group completers: 6/10 cCBT group showed significant improvement on 7/10 subscales compared with control group, which showed significant improvement on only three subscales
(Wuthrich et al. 2012)	"Cool Teens" eight sessions thirty minutes CD-Rom Brief telephone support with therapist	Age fourteen to seventeen Community/referred sample Primary diagnosis of anxiety disorder n = 43	RCT	Post-treatment—41% in intervention group no longer met diagnostic criteria for primary diagnosis. At three-month follow-up 23.5% no longer met diagnostic criteria for primary diagnosis

Source: Adapted from Richardson et al., 2010.

(Storch et al. 2011) randomly assigned to either web-camera CBT (W-CBT) (sixteen participants) or a waitlist control group (fifteen participants) found that W-CBT was superior to the control group in all primary outcome measures with a large effect size (Cohen's d >1.36). Eighty-one percent of the W-CBT group were treatment responders, and 56 percent were in remission (compared to 13 percent treatment responders and 13 percent in remission in the control group). The authors highlight the potential benefits of this intervention to overcome potential barriers in treatment dissemination.

A review of the use of virtual reality in the assessment and treatment of OCD highlighted the potential for this technology to perform interventions such as exposure-response prevention (Kim et al., 2009). The virtual reality allows a more controlled, consistent, and objectively measurable intervention compared to imagery work and yet is not as aversive as in vivo experiences. However, this approach has not been evaluated.

Somatic Disorders

Chronic Fatigue Syndrome

One technology-based program for the treatment of adolescents with chronic fatigue syndrome has been described: the trial of an internet-based program for adolescents called "Fatigue in Teenagers on the interNET (FITNET)" which was based on a cognitive behavioral model previously used in the treatment of adolescents and their families (Nijhof et al., 2012). There were three elements to the program: email consultations, termed e-consults, between the adolescent and a trained therapist; online psycho-educational material; and twenty-one interactive cognitive behavioral modules. Parents followed a similar program of psycho-education and CBT modules but with less detailed information than the patient. The FITNET group was compared to a group receiving "treatment as usual" on school attendance, fatigue, and physical functioning at six and twelve months. The FITNET group showed improvement in all measures with significantly higher school attendance compared to the TAU group. Improvement in the FITNET group was sustained at twelve months. The thirty-two patients who had not recovered after six months of TAU crossed over to the FITNET arm and had similar outcomes to the primary FITNET group at twelve months. The FITNET group benefited from early treatment due to the reduced barriers to therapy inherent to chronic fatigue.

Eating Disorders

There have been four approaches in the development of technology for treating eating disorders. These included using videoconferencing (Goldfield and Boachie, 2003; Mitchell et al., 2008) and email-based therapy (Robinson and Serfaty, 2008) to improve access to interventions such as family therapy. CD-ROM (Schmidt et al., 2008) and web-based therapy (ter Huurne et al., 2013; Pretorius et al., 2009) programs for treating eating disorders, primarily in those with binge eating behaviors or bulimia, have been described.

Virtual reality has been used in the treatment of eating disorders since the 1990s and a recent review (Ferrer-Garcia, Gutiérrez-Maldonado and Riva, 2013) summarizes the published work in this area which they conclude has been largely undertaken by two groups: Riva and colleagues in Italy, and Perpina, Botella, and Banos in Spain. It has been used in combination with traditional cognitive approaches and appears particularly effective at addressing body image disturbance. A key factor appears to be the manipulation of perspective in virtual reality allowing a person to experience a scenario from different viewpoints—seeing and thinking about themselves differently. No published trials have been identified using virtual reality specifically with adolescents or children; it is an area in need of future research.

Autistic Spectrum Disorders

Developmental disorders frequently require interventions that are not aimed at recovery but at skill building. Therefore, improved coping and quality of life interventions for these disorders take the form of "training packages" rather than "treatment."

Young people with autistic spectrum disorders (ASD) find it more difficult to develop social skills, particularly making use of non-verbal cues, such as body posture and facial expression. Addressing these difficulties and trying to enhance the skills of young people with ASD has been the aim of several different uses of technology over the last two decades. The approaches developed in the late 1990s used virtual reality and more recently tele-practice, computer-based, and computer-game based interventions. A challenge for technology is that there is a perceived difficulty in children with ASD to generalize learning from one environment to other areas or situations in their lives.

More recently an interactive avatar-based social skills program has been developed (Hopkins et al., 2011). It aimed to develop a realistic interaction between the young person and the software to help them develop emotion- and face-recognition skills. It includes a series of games based on current understanding of how and why those with ASD have difficulty with social interactions. A randomized controlled study which separated young people into high- and low-functioning groups, with a control group for each, was conducted. Both high- and low-functioning groups showed significant increase in total emotion-recognition skills compared to their respective control groups. The authors highlight that young people found the computer software acceptable and reportedly found it enjoyable. There were noted additional benefits for a small number of students in that using the training software improved their computer skills.

Google SketchUp, a 3D graphic design package, has been reported to be very useful in enabling children on the autistic spectrum to express themselves and improve their social skills. As a result of this feedback from customers Google set up "Project Spectrum" to help further develop the use of SketchUp for children with ASD. A small group of children with high-functioning autism who were involved in a workshop to enhance family interaction across generations using Google SketchUp has been investigated and evaluation of this approach is awaited (Wright et al., 2012).

Neuropsychiatric Disorders

Attention Deficit and Hyperactivity Disorder (ADHD)

Parenting interventions represent the main approach to non-pharmacological treatment of ADHD. Recent developments include delivery methods that use digital technology. Early attempts to use technology involved disseminating materials for self-directed interventions through videotapes (Webster-Stratton, 1994). CD-ROMs and laser discs were subsequently developed and added to the potential for interactivity (Lagges and Gordon, 1999).

Sanders et al. (2008) published a study using a combination of a UK broadcast television documentary showing five families undergoing a Triple P program (Sanders, Turner, Markie-Dadds, 2002) as well as providing additional material in the form of a self-help workbook, web-based information with audio-visual content, reminders about episodes, and email support to families. This "enhanced" program was compared to a group who received no additional support and just watched the television program. They found that those with enhanced support showed greater improvement in the child's behavior, improvement on two of three parenting measures, and greater overall satisfaction. The web-based materials were accessed frequently, particularly at the beginning of the series. There was low level use of the email support with improvement related to the number of TV episodes viewed. Overall there was a lower completion rate than seen with face-to-face interventions.

A feasibility study of web-based Parent-Adolescent Conflict Training (PACT) for families with teenagers with ADHD has been tested against only two of the twelve modules included in the package (Carpenter et al., 2004). Qualitative data indicates parental satisfaction but a full evaluation of this web-based package is required.

Traumatic Brain Injury

Following traumatic brain injury (TBI) in childhood, psychiatric problems are common and debilitating. Wade et al. (2009) developed a web-based intervention, "Internet-based Interacting Together Everyday, Recovery After Childhood TBI (I-INTERACT)," which used Parent-Child Interaction Therapy (PCIT) as its therapeutic model with the aim of improving rehabilitation outcomes and overcoming barriers of time, distance, and transportation. The web-based program was delivered through ten core and five supplemental sessions and contained material presented through video, text, and guided activity. After completing the self-guided session parent had a fifty-minute video conference session with a trained therapist. Part of this session would involve live coaching using a webcam and a Bluetooth headset that enabled the therapist to talk to the parent without the child's awareness. Following a feasibility study with nine families they reported promising results with significant increases in positive parenting skills and a decrease in negative parenting behaviors. The program was generally well received by families though reported barriers included technical difficulty with lack of an internet connection strong enough to support the video conference, too much choice about when to complete the modules so a tendency to put them off, and frequent house moves. A randomized control trial of this package is currently under way (http://clinicaltrials.gov/show/NCT01214694).

Psychotic Disorders

Psychotic disorders include schizophrenia, delusional disorder, acute and transient psychotic disorders, schizoaffective disorder, and bipolar disorder. Many sufferers of severe mental illness become socially withdrawn or isolated making engagement with and maintaining regular contact with mental health services more difficult. Technology holds promise in overcoming these difficulties. Technology-based interventions have included using mobile phone messaging, mobile applications, internet- and computer-based programs, and virtual reality. There is some evidence for these interventions in young people.

Preliminary evidence from studies with adults suggests that SMS-based intervention can be used to monitor early warning signs (Spaniel et al., 2008), improve medication adherence, socialization, and auditory hallucinations (Granholm et al., 2012). Three approaches to using mobile phones with adults have been described (Depp et al., 2010). These "proof of concept" studies involve automating interventions: prompting engagement in personalized self-management behaviors based on real-time data; employing experience sampling via text messages to facilitate case management; and a third approach which builds on group functional skills training by incorporating between-session mobile phone contact with therapists.

As seen in other disorders this use of technology is an additional means of communication within existing models of care designed to enhance engagement and treatment compliance. Others have used technology to develop entirely new models of care that would not otherwise be possible. Alverez-Jimenez et al. reported the development of a novel model of behavioral intervention called "Moderated Online Social Therapy" or "MOST" (Alvarez-Jimenez et al. 2013). They described the features in this way: "The MOST model integrates: i) peer-to-peer online social networking; ii) individually tailored interactive psychosocial interventions; and (iii) involvement of expert mental health and peer moderators to ensure the safety of the intervention" (p.145). From this theoretical framework they developed the "HORYZONS" program, an online psychosocial intervention designed as an intermediate step of care between specialist services and standard care in the treatment of first-episode psychosis. A pilot study to test the feasibility, acceptability, safety, and potential clinical utility of the HORYZONS program was carried out with twenty participants aged fifteen to twenty-five years old from an Early Intervention in Psychosis Centre in Melbourne, Australia. They reported that the majority of participants felt "safe, empowered and more socially connected using HORYZONS"; there was also significant reduction in depressive symptoms at four-week follow-up. Acknowledging the limitations of this initial study the authors conclude that it demonstrates a proof of concept and planned further evaluations of the program for maintaining the specialized treatment effects.

DISCUSSION

There is evidence that digital technology in various forms is increasingly being used effectively to prevent and ameliorate psychological distress and disorder in children and adolescents. The systematic evaluation of these interventions is in the early stages with only a small number of published randomized trials. Digital technology has been used to directly deliver therapy (e.g., internet-based groups and virtual reality), to enhance the delivery of therapy between a live therapist and patient (e.g., video conferencing), to increase the ability for a patient and clinician to monitor and manage symptoms without the barriers of time and space (e.g., asynchronous mobile messaging or email), and to deliver interventions with less need for direct professional involvement (e.g., computerized CBT) .

Published research in the field of technology-based interventions range from descriptions of novel practices, small case series, and feasibility studies to randomized control trials. Most papers reveal generally positive findings, though methodologically rigorous studies are currently scarce. A recurrent weakness of the RCTs is the poor selection of control groups. These groups were commonly treatment as usual or waiting list control and only in a few cases do the control groups use an equivalent face-to-face intervention. Where direct comparisons were made with an equivalent existing, non-technology-based approach, the studies looked for non-inferiority of the technology-based interventions. A further difficulty accurately evaluating the effectiveness was the poor completion rate for modules or specific tasks.

Most of the trials reported were conducted by the program developers. This lack of independent evaluation leads to potential bias in the description of results and reporting the acceptability of these programs. Many clinicians view their engagement and relationship with the patient as critical to their work and struggle with the idea of loss of face-to-face contact; integrating technological packages into their work might prove difficult. Broad dissemination therefore remains largely unevaluated.

Overcoming Barriers

Two themes recur within the evidence base. Firstly, using digital technology to provide management, treatment, or prevention was viewed as "cheaper" than traditional forms of intervention in terms of both professional time and other resources. While technological interventions are viewed as cheaper, there is significant cost involved in developing, distributing, and maintaining technology-based interventions, raising the question about who bares this cost. Formal health economic evaluations are lacking, and it is not clear that there are cost savings from using technology.

The second theme is the acceptability of the technology to young people and their families. The everyday familiarity with mobile phones and computers might contribute to the widely reported finding that technology-based interventions are highly acceptable to young people and their families. Using technology might be less anxiety provoking than consulting a mental health professional. Many of the interventions are not limited to "office hours" and can be accessed at the control of the young person at a time that suits them, presenting as less disruptive or intrusive to young people's lives. Since the internet is constantly functioning, interventions using internet-based communication have the potential to be constantly available and not restricted by traditional models of working hours (Alvarez-Jimenez et al., 2013).

The ability to start interventions more quickly was seen as a further advantage. Professional limitations on capacity could be reduced using these interventions which offers promise in terms of closing the widely recognised gap in treatment availability for children and young people. It may prevent deterioration in the condition of those who might otherwise be subject to long waiting times. This is particularly valid for computer-based, self-directed interventions. Where clinicians remain involved, technology increases the clinician's capacity to engage in therapeutic work with more patients simultaneously.

The internet also allows mass social, interactive communication. This capacity has only been exploited in a handful of programs across disorders through the use of chat rooms or more sophisticated platforms such as that in the HORYZONS study (Alvarez-Jimenez et al., 2013). A common finding was the need for expert moderation of these shared internet therapeutic environments. Working with groups is not new territory for therapists in CAMHS, but moderating groups across a virtual environment may be more challenging. Further difficulties around creating social therapeutic environments will be discussed later.

Technology-based interventions offer opportunities to overcome barriers integral to the disorders. The FITNET trial highlighted this with the treatment of chronic fatigue syndrome using remotely accessed care. Anxiety disorders which prevent young people accessing clinic-based services are also disorders which might be helped with these approaches.

New Frontiers

The developers of the HORYZONS program have taken digital interventions a step further in terms of using the social capacity of the internet. Rather than taking existing therapy models such as cognitive behavioral therapy, the model starts with the ecology of the online social environment and tries to adapt its processes to develop a new model of therapeutic interaction. This innovative approach may yield further creative applications in the future; virtual realities, using sophisticated characters with which users interact, are already being created. Within the gaming world, technology that enables others to interact and network in similar virtually created fantasy worlds is widely available and enjoyed in massive multiplayer online role-playing games (MMORPGS) such as *World of Warcraft*. It is possible that as part of prevention or treatment, the interaction between users could be extended beyond the two-dimensional chat forum to a group therapy approach carried out using avatars in a 3D virtual reality.

The use of game play is already a common theme across computer-based or internet-based programs. The use of game play in non-gaming activities, such as CBT, is known as gamification and is an area of increasing development in business' digital strategy. Child and adolescent use of computer games is ubiquitous, and gaming is moving from computers and gaming consoles to handheld devices such as tablet computers and smartphones as ownership of these devices increases. The low rates of completing therapeutic interventions, particular those involving gamification of the delivery, compared with those of traditional computer games suggests mental health intervention developers should work more closely with traditional game designers to improve the attractiveness of such packages.

Most technology-based interventions report that a team is involved in the development. They include the following: clinicians, educational specialists, hardware developers, computer programers, health informatics experts, web and graphic designers, and young people and their families. This co-constructed digital multidisciplinary team approach to the development of technology-based therapeutic systems, with iterative use of focus groups and testing, is a divergence from the historical model of clinician experience and insight informed development of interventions. Furthermore, technology-based interventions might shift the nature of care from a more paternalistic, clinician-lead model of therapy to a co-authored or patient-lead model.

The geographical barriers to providing mental health services to young people and their families might be overcome by the use of technology. There might no longer be a need for young people to travel potentially large distances from remote or rural areas to urban areas where specialists are concentrated to access care (Hilt et al., 2013). Where there are socio-cultural values that increase reluctance to engage with mental health services this could also be overcome by the ability to access care remotely through technology without the potential stigmatizing difficulties of attending a mental health clinic.

Technology-based programs are likely to lead to opportunities for alternative service designs. Remote monitoring of symptoms and treatment provision might allow wider provision at lower cost and free up human resources to attend to the most severe cases. A tiered approach from self-directed computer packages, to instant-messaging-delivered therapy, video-linked sessions, virtual reality, and finally face-to-face contact, with a mix of individual and moderated social network approaches, could create more flexibility in a service to meet the needs of their population compared to current service models.

The need for confidentiality within technology-based approaches brings new challenges. Improving confidentiality during the process of information transfer has occurred through the use of portal sites that allow not only the provision of self-help materials but also communication with professionals via both synchronous and asynchronous messaging functions. These sites require separate logins for each user and allow the interactions between a young person and their parents to be kept private and separate where appropriate. Portal sites are run from centrally located, secure mainframe servers where data is stored. This reduces the potential for data to be intercepted or disrupted as it never leaves the protected processes of the mainframe servers. The need for such sophisticated confidentiality and data security may limit the potential for programs to be developed and disseminated without the backing of large organisations, such as university medical centers, that already have access to secure IT facilities.

CONCLUSION

The integration of technology into everyday life is increasing rapidly. In parallel, the integration of treatment interventions and prevention programs within child and adolescent mental health holds great potential. Many current researchers and clinicians are challenged by the need to effectively incorporate these approaches, but it would appear that technology has the potential to significantly ameliorate and prevent mental health problems in young people.

REFERENCES

Abeles, P., Verduyn, C., Robinson, A., Smith, P., Yule, W., and Proudfoot, J. "Computerized CBT for Adolescent Depression (stressbusters) and Its Initial Evaluation through an Extended Case Series." *Behavioral and Cognitive Psychotherapy* 37 (2009):151–65.

Alvarez-Jimenez, M., Bendall, S., Lederman, R., Wadley, G., Chinnery, G., Vargas, S., Larkin, M., Killackey, E., McGorry, P. D., and Gleeson, J. F. "On the HORYZON: Moderated Online Social Therapy for Long-term Recovery in First Episode Psychosis." *Schizophrenia Research* 143 (2013):143–49.

Andersson, E., Ljotsson, B., Hedman, E., Kaldo, V., Paxling, B., Andersson, G., Lindefors, N., and Ruck, C. "Internet-based Cognitive Behavior Therapy for Obsessive Compulsive Disorder: A Pilot Study." *BMC Psychiatry* 11 (2011).

Calear, A. L, Christensen, H., Mackinnon, A., Griffiths, K. M. and O'Kearney, R. "The YouthMood Project: A Cluster Randomized Controlled Trial of an Online Cognitive Behavioral Program with Adolescents." *Journal of Consulting and Clinical Psychology* 77 (2009):1021–32.

Carpenter, Erika M., Fred Frankel, Michael Marina, Naihua Duan, and Susan L. Smalley. 2004. "Internet Treatment Delivery of Parent-Adolescent Conflict Training for Families with an ADHD Teen: A Feasibility Study." *Child & Family Behavior Therapy* 26 (3):1–20.

Depp, C. A., Mausbach, B., Granholm, E., Cardenas V., Ben-Zeev, D., Patterson, T. L, Lebowitz, B. D., and Jeste, D. V. "Mobile Interventions for Severe Mental Illness: Design and Preliminary Data from Three Approaches." *The Journal of Nervous and Mental Disease* 198 (2010):715–21.

Ferrer-Garcia, M., Gutiérrez-Maldonado, J. and Riva, G. "Virtual Reality Based Treatments in Eating Disorders and Obesity: A Review." *Journal of Contemporary Psychotherapy* (June 2013):1–33.

Gerrits, R. S., van der Zanden, R. A., Visscher, R. F., and Conijn. B. P. "Master Your Mood Online: A Preventive Chat Group Intervention for Adolescents." *Advances in Mental Health* 6 (2007):152–62.

Goldfield, S., and Boachie, A. "Delivery of Family Therapy in the Treatment of Anorexia Nervosa Using Telehealth." *Telemedicine Journal and e-Health* 9 (2003):111–14.

Granholm, E., Ben-Zeev, D., Link, P. C., Bradshaw, K. R., and Holden, J. L. "Mobile Assessment and Treatment for Schizophrenia (MATS): A Pilot Trial of an Interactive Text-messaging Intervention for Medication Adherence, Socialization, and Auditory Hallucinations." *Schizophrenia Bulletin* 38 (2012):414–25.

Hakak, R., and Szeftel, R. "Clinical Use of Telemedicine in Child Psychiatry." *FOCUS: The Journal of Lifelong Learning in Psychiatry* 6 (2008):293–96.

Hilt, R. J., Romaire, M. A., McDonell, M. G., Sears, J. M., Krupski, A., Thompson, J. N., Myers J., Trupin, E. W. "The Partnership Access Line: Evaluating a Child Psychiatry Consult Program in Washington State." *JAMA Pediatrics* 167 (2013):162–68.

Hopkins, I. M., Gower, W., Perez, A., Smith, S., Amthor, R., Wimsatt, F. C., and Biasini, J. "Avatar Assistant: Improving Social Skills in Students with an ASD through a Computer-based Intervention." *Journal of Autism and Developmental Disorders* 41 (2011):1543–55.

Kauer, S. D., Reid, S. R., Dale Crooke, A. H., Khor, A., Hearps, S. J. C., Jorm, A. F., Sanci, L., Patton, G. "Self-Monitoring Using Mobile Phones in the Early Stages of Adolescent Depression: Randomized Controlled Trial." *Journal of Medical Internet Research* 14 (2012).

Kim, K., Kim, C-H., Kim, S-Y,. Roh, D., and Kim, S. I. "Virtual Reality for Obsessive-compulsive Disorder: Past and the Future." *Psychiatry Investigation* 6 (2009):115–21.

Klein, B., Mitchell, J., Gilson K., Shandley, K., Austin, D., Kiropoulos, L., Abbott, J., and Cannard, G. "A Therapist Assisted Internet Based CBT Intervention for Posttraumatic Stress Disorder: Preliminary Results." *Cognitive Behavior Therapy* 38 (2009):121–31.

Lagges, A. M., and Gordon, D. A. "Use of an Interactive Laserdisc Parent Training Program with Teenage Parents." *Child & Family Behavior Therapy* 21 (1999):19–37.

Lefebvre, R. C., and Bornkessel, A. S. "Digital Social Networks and Health." *Circulation* 127 (2013):1829–36.

Lovell, K, and Bee, P. "Optimising Treatment Resources for OCD: A Review of the Evidence Base for Technology-enhanced Delivery." *Journal of Mental Health* 20 (2011):525–42.

March, S., Spence, S. H., and Donovan, C. L. "The Efficacy of an Internet-based Cognitive-behavioral Therapy Intervention for Child Anxiety Disorders." *Journal of Pediatric Psychology* 34 (2009):474–87.

Matthews, M., and Doherty, G. "In the Mood: Engaging Teenagers in Psychotherapy Using Mobile Phones." CHI'11 Proceedings of the SIGCHI Conference on Human Factors in Computing System (2011):2947–56.

Merry, S. N., Stasiak, K., Shepherd, M., Frampton, C., Fleming, T., and Lucassen, M. F. G. "The Effectiveness of SPARX, a Computerised Self Help Intervention for Adolescents Seeking Help for Depression: Randomized Controlled Non-inferiority Trial." *BMJ* 344 (2012):e2598–e2598.

Mitchell, J. E., Crosby, R. D., Wonderlich, S. A., Crow, S., Lancaster, K., Simonich, H., Swan-Kremeier, L., Lysne, C., and Cook Myers, T. "A Randomized Trial Comparing the Efficacy of Cognitive–behavioral Therapy for Bulimia Nervosa Delivered via Telemedicine Versus Face-to-face." *Behavior Research and Therapy* 46 (2008):581–92.

Mundt, J. C., Emslie G. J., Reyes, T., Mayes, T. L., Joyner. K, and King, J. "Assessing Feasibility, Reliability, and Validity of Computer-automated Interactive Sms Text Messages to Self-report Depression Symptoms in Children and Adolescents Using the Quick Inventory of Depressive Symptomatology-Adolescent." *Journal of Child and Adolescent Psychopharmacology* 21 (2011).

Nelson, E-L., Barnard, M., and Cain, S. "Treating Childhood Depression over Videoconferencing." *Telemedicine Journal and E-health: The Official Journal of the American Telemedicine Association* 9 (2003):49–55.

Nijhof, L., Bleijenberg G., Uiterwaal S. P. M., Kimpen L. L., and van Elise, M. "Effectiveness of Internet-based Cognitive Behavioral Treatment for Adolescents with Chronic Fatigue Syndrome (FITNET): A Randomized Controlled Trial." *Lancet* 379 (2012):141–218.

O'Kearney, R., Gibson, M., Christensen, H., and Griffiths, K. M. "Effects of a Cognitive-behavioral Internet Program on Depression, Vulnerability to Depression and Stigma in Adolescent Males: A School-based Controlled Trial." *Cognitive Behavior Therapy* 35 (2006):43–54.

O'Kearney, R., Kang, K., Christensen, H., and Griffiths, K. "A Controlled Trial of a School-based Internet Program for Reducing Depressive Symptoms in Adolescent Girls." *Depression and Anxiety* 26 (2009):65–72.

Pretorius, N., Arcelus, J., Beecham, J., Dawson, H., Doherty, F., Eisler, I.,Gallagher, C., Gowers, S., Isaacs, G., Johnson-Sabine, E., Jones, A., Newell, C., Morris, J., Richards, L., Ringwood, S., Rowlands, L., Simic, M., Treasure, J., Waller, G., Williams, C., Yi, I., Yoshioka, M., and Schmidt, U. "Cognitive-Behavioral Therapy for Adolescents with Bulimic Symptomatology: The Acceptability and Effectiveness of Internet-based Delivery." *Behavior Research and Therapy* 47 (2009):729–36.

Richardson, T., Stallard, P., and Vellenian, S. "Computerized Congnitive Behavioral Therapy for the Prevention and Treatment of Depression and Anxiety in Children and Adolescents: A Systematic Review." *Clinical Child and Family Psychology Review* 13 (3) (2010): 275–90.

Rizzo, A., John, B., Newman, B., Williams, J., Hartholt, A., Lethin, C., and Buckwalter, G. J. "Virtual Reality as a Tool for Delivering PTSD Exposure Therapy and Stress Resilience Training." *Military Behavioral Health* 1 (1) (2013):52–58.

Robinson, P., and Serfaty, M. "Getting Better Byte by Byte: A Pilot Randomized Controlled Trial of Email Therapy for Bulimia Nervosa and Binge Eating Disorder." *European Eating Disorders Review* 16 (2008):84–93.

Sanders, M. R., Turner, K. M. T., and Markie-Dadds, C. "The Development and Dissemination of the Triple P—Positive Parenting Program: A Multilevel, Evidence-based System of Parenting and Family Support." *Prevention Science* 3 (3) (2002):173–89.

Sanders, M., Calam, R., Durand, M., Liversidge, T., and Carmont, S. A. "Does Self-directed and Web-based Support for Parents Enhance the Effects of Viewing a Reality Television Series Based on the Triple P—Positive Parenting Program?" *Journal of Child Psychology and Psychiatry* 49 (2008):924–32.

Schmidt, U., Andiappan, M., Grover, M., Robinson, S., Perkins, S., Dugmore, O., Treasure, J., Landau, S., Eisler, I., and Williams, C. "Randomized Controlled Trial of CD-ROM-based Cognitive-Behavioral Self-care for Bulimia Nervosa." *The British Journal of Psychiatry* 193 (2008):493–500.

Shandley, K., Austin, D., Klein, B., and Kyrios, M. "An Evaluation of 'Reach Out Central': An Online Gaming Program for Supporting the Mental Health of Young People." *Health Education Research* 25 (2010):563–74.

Spaniel, F., Vohlídka, P., Kozeny, J., Novák, T., Hrdlicka, J., Motlova, L., Cermák, J., and Höschl, C. "The Information Technology Aided Relapse Prevention Program in Schizophrenia: An Extension of a Mirror-design Follow-up." *International Journal of Clinical Practice* 62 (2008):1943–47.

Spence, S. H., Donovan, C. L., March, S., Gamble, A., Anderson, R. E, Prosser, S., and Kenardy, J. "A Randomized Controlled Trial of Online Versus Clinic-based CBT for Adolescent Anxiety." *Journal of Consulting and Clinical Psychology* 79 (2011):629–42.

Spence, S. H., Holmes, J. M., March, S., and Lipp, O. V. "The Feasibility and Outcome of Clinic Plus Internet Delivery of Cognitive-Behavior Therapy for Childhood Anxiety." *Journal of Consulting and Clinical Psychology* 74 (2006):614–21.

Stallard, P., Richardson, T., Velleman, S., and Attwood, M. "Computerized CBT (Think, Feel, Do) for Depression and Anxiety in Children and Adolescents: Outcomes and Feedback from a Pilot Randomized Controlled Trial." *Behavioral and Cognitive Psychotherapy* 39 (2011):273–84.

Storch, E. A., Caporino, N. E., Morgan, J. R., Lewin, A. B., Rojas, A., Brauer, L., Larson, M. J., and Murphy, T. K. "Preliminary Investigation of Web-camera Delivered Cognitive-behavioral Therapy for Youth with Obsessive-compulsive Disorder." *Psychiatry Research* 189 (2011):407–12.

ter Huurne, E. D., Postel M. G., de Haan, H., Drossaert, C. H. C., and DeJong, C. J. "Web-based Treatment Program Using Intensive Therapeutic Contact for Patients with Eating Disorders: Before-after Study." *Journal of Medical Internet Research* 15 (2013).

Turner, C., Heyman, I., Futh, A., & Lovell, K. "A Pilot Study of Telephone Behavioral Therapy for Obsessive-Compulsive Disorder in Young People." *Behavioral and Cognitive Psychotherapy* 37 (2009):469–74.

Van der Zanden, R., Kramer J., Gerrits, R., and Cuijpers, P. "Effectiveness of an Online Group Course for Depression in Adolescents and Young Adults: A Randomized Trial." *Journal of Medical Internet Research* (2012).

Van Voorhees, B. W., Fogel, J., Reinecke, M., Gladstone, T., Stuart, S., Gollan, J., Bradford, N., et al. "Randomized Clinical Trial of an Internet-based Depression Prevention Program for Adolescents (Project CATCH-IT) in Primary Care: 12-week Outcomes." *Journal of Developmental and Behavioral Pediatrics* 30 (2009):23–37.

Van Voorhees, B. W., Vanderplough-Booth, K., Fogel, J., Gladstone, T., Bell, C., Stuart, S., Gollan, J., et al."Integrative Internet-based Depression Prevention for Adolescents: A Randomized Clinical Trial in Primary Care for Vulnerability and Protective Factors." *Journal of the Canadian Academy of Child and Adolescent Psychiatry* 17 (2008):184–96.

Wade, S. L., Oberjohn, K., Burkhardt, A., and Greenberg, I. "Feasibility and Preliminary Efficacy of a Web-based Parenting Skills Program for Young Children with Traumatic Brain Injury." *The Journal of Head Trauma Rehabilitation* 24 (2009):239–47.

Walshe, D. G., Lewis, E. J., Kim, S. I., O'Sullivan, K., and Wiederhold, B. K. "Exploring the Use of Computer Games and Virtual Reality in Exposure Therapy for Fear of Driving Following a Motor Vehicle Accident." *CyberPsychology & Behavior* 6 (3) (2003):329–34.

Webster-Stratton, C. "Advancing Videotape Parent Training: A Comparison Study." *Journal of Consulting and Clinical Psychology* 62 (3) (1994):583.

Wright, C., Diener, M., Dunn, L., and Wright, S. "Enhancing Family Connections via Technology (Google SketchUp) for Children with Autism Spectrum Disorders." *Journal of Intellectual Disability Research* 56 (7–8) (2012).

Wuthrich, V. M., Rapee, R. M., Cunningham, M. J., Lyneham, H. J., Hudson, J. L., and Schniering, C. A. "A Randomized Controlled Trial of the Cool Teens CD-ROM Computerized Program for Adolescent Anxiety." *Journal of the American Academy of Child Adolescent Psychiatry* 51 (3) (2012):261–70.

Index

About the Contributors

Adeyinka M. Akinsulure-Smith, PhD, is a licensed psychologist originally from Sierra Leone. She is assistant professor in the Department of Psychology at City College of the City University of New York. She has extensive clinical experience working with war trauma survivors, refugees, asylees and asylum seekers, survivors of sexual violence, persons afflicted with and affected by HIV/AIDS, and culturally diverse populations. Dr. Akinsulure-Smith has been conducting individual and group psychotherapy as well as psychological assessments with clients in the Bellevue/NYU Program for Survivors of Torture since 1999. She has been involved in human rights investigations in Sierra Leone with Physicians for Human Rights and the United Nations Mission in Sierra Leone, Human Rights Division.

Anne E. Becker, MD, PhD, is the Maude and Lillian Presley Professor of Global Health and Social Medicine at Harvard Medical School, where she also serves as vice chair of the Department of Global Health and Social Medicine. An anthropologist and psychiatrist, Dr. Becker has combined ethnographic, other qualitative, and epidemiologic methods in her research to focus on the impact of social and cultural environment on mental health. She is the author of *Body, Self, and Society: The View from Fiji*, which probes the cultural mediation of self-agency and body experience. More recently, Dr. Becker's NIMH-funded research has investigated the impact of rapid economic and social transition on eating pathology, suicide, and other youth health risk behaviors in Fiji. Presently, with NIMH and Fogarty International Center support, she and co-PI Pere Eddy Eustache of Zanmi Lasante are conducting a mental health research capacity building project and novel school-based youth mental health pilot intervention in central Haiti. Dr. Becker is the former director of the Eating Disorders Clinical and Research Program at Massachusetts General Hospital, past president of the Academy for Eating Disorders, and served as a member of the American Psychiatric Association's DSM-5 Eating Disorders Work Group. She is past coeditor in chief of the journal, *Culture, Medicine and Psychiatry*, and is presently an associate editor of the *International Journal of Eating Disorders*. Dr. Becker is the 2013 recipient of the Price Family Award for Research Excellence from the National Eating Disorders Association.

Dr. Becker received her bachelor's degree in anthropology from Harvard College, summa cum laude. She received her medical training at Harvard Medical School and received a doctoral degree in anthropology from the Harvard Graduate School of Arts & Sciences as part of a joint MD-PhD program in social sciences supported by the MacArthur Foundation. She also received a master of science degree in epidemiology from the Harvard School of Public Health. Dr. Becker completed her residency in the Department of Psychiatry at the Massachusetts General Hospital in 1994.

Nicolas Berthelot, PhD, Centre de recherche de l'Institut universitaire en santé mentale de Québec, Canada, Département des sciences infirmières, Université du Québec à Trois-Rivières, Canada.

Theresa S. Betancourt, ScD, MA, is associate professor of child health and human rights in the Department of Global Health and Population at the Harvard School of Public Health and director of the Research Program on Children and Global Adversity (RPCGA). Her central research interests include the developmental and psychosocial consequences of concentrated adversity on children and families, resilience and protective processes in child and adolescent mental health, refugee families, and applied cross-cultural mental health research. She is principal investigator of a prospective longitudinal study of war-affected youth in Sierra Leone and has developed and is evaluating the impact of a Family Strengthening Intervention for HIV-affected children and families in Rwanda. She has written extensively on mental health and resilience in children facing adversity including recent articles in *Child Development, Journal of the American Academy of Child and Adolescent Psychiatry, Social Science and Medicine, and PLOS One.*

Huey-Ling Chiang, MD, is a visiting child and adolescent psychiatrist in the Department of Psychiatry, Far-eastern Memorial Hospital, Taipei County, Taiwan, and adjunct instructer and visiting psychiatrist, Department of Psychiatry, National Taiwan University Hospital and College of Medicine, Taipei, Taiwan. She received her MD from National Yangming University and is currently pursuing her PhD at the Graduate Institute of Clinical Medicine, National Taiwan University, under the direction of Professor Susan S.-F. Gau.

Anne-Claire Crombag is in psychiatric training in The Hague and Leiden, in the Netherlands.

Susan Shur-Fen Gau, MD, PhD, is director/chair of the Department of Psychiatry, National Taiwan University Hospital (NTUH) and College of Medicine, Taipei, Taiwan, and professor of psychiatry, epidemiology, psychology, occupational therapy, clinical medicine, and brain and mind sciences, National Taiwan University. She received her MD from Chun-Shan Medical University and a PhD in epidemiology from Yale University, and received psychiatry training at NTUH. Her current research interests are clinical, neuropsychological, electrophysiological, neuroimaging, pharmacoepidemiology, and genetic studies on ADHD and autism.

E. Gilbert, PhD, Centre de recherche de l'Institut universitaire en santé mentale de Québec, Canada.

Katrina Hann, BSc, MA, is a public health research professional with over four years' experience working in academic partnerships for global health research in low-resource settings in sub-Saharan Africa. She has specific interests in capacity building for health research, cross-cultural mental health, and the ethics of conducting research with vulnerable populations. Nathan Hansen, Department of Psychiatry, Yale School of Medicine, New Haven, USA.

Nathan Hansen, PhD, is associate professor in the College of Public Health at the University of Georgia. His research focuses on the intersection of mental health, traumatic stress, and substance use. He has considerable experience in intervention development and cultural adaptation and has served as an investigator on numerous intervention development studies domestically and internationally.

Jian-Ping He, MSc, is a statistician of the Genetic Epidemiology Branch in the Intramural Research Program at the National Institute of Mental Health (NIMH). Ms. He received a bachelor's degree in medicine from Shanghai Medical University in China. She received a master's degree in biostatistics from Shanghai Medical University and a master's degree in science, majoring in epidemiology, from Michigan State University. She is the chief analyst for large-scale epidemiologic studies at the NIMH Intramural Research Program and has played a leading role in facilitating the dissemination of the first U.S. national studies on child mental health including the National Comorbidity Survey (NCS) –Replication (NCS-R) and its adolescent extension (NCS-R) and the National Health and Nutrition Examination Survey (NHANES). She has received awards from the NIMH director for her contribution to an epidemiologic study of the U.S. military and from Kelly Services for excellence and productivity in epidemiologic analyses.

Matthew Hodes, MBBS, BSc, MSc, PhD, FRCPsych, is senior lecturer in child and adolescent psychiatry at Imperial College London and honorary consultant in child and adolescent psychiatry in CNWL NHS Trust. His research interests include migration and cultural influences on mental health and service utilization and the interface of physical and mental health in young people.

Miki Igarashi, Showa University, Karasuyama Hospital, Tokyo, Japan.

Nobumasa Kato, MD, PhD, Department of Psychiatry, Showa University Karasuyama Hospital, JST CREST, Tokyo, Japan.

Soo-Yung Kim, MD, National Rehabilitation Center for Persons with Disabilities, Saitama, Japan.

Henrikje Klasen is an anthropologist and child and adolescent psychiatrist who trained in London (LSE and Maudsley) and now works as head of psychiatric training and associate professor in Leiden and The Haague, in the Netherlands.

Arthur Kleinman, MD (born March 11, 1941), is a physician and anthropologist who is now in his thirty-seventh year at Harvard. A graduate of Stanford University and Stanford Medical School, with an MA in social anthropology from Harvard and trained in psychiatry at the Massachusetts General Hospital, Kleinman is a leading figure in several fields: medical anthropology, cultural psychiatry, global health, social medicine, and medical humanities. He has conducted research in China from 1978 to the present, and in Taiwan from 1969 until 1978. In 1973 he taught Harvard's first course in medical anthropology, and in 1982 he inaugurated Harvard's PhD program in medical anthropology.

He has supervised more than seventy-five PhD students and over two hundred postdoctoral fellows. He has also taught generations of Harvard undergraduates, medical students, MA students, and residents. Kleinman is the author of six books, coauthor of two others, coeditor of nearly thirty volumes and eight special issues of journals, and author of over 300 articles, book chapters, reviews, and introductions. Kleinman is a member of the Institute of Medicine of the National Academies and the American Academy of Arts and Sciences. The 2001 winner of the Franz Boas Award of the American Anthropological Association (its highest award), Kleinman is a Distinguished Lifetime Fellow of the American Psychiatric Association. He has twice given the distinguished lecture at NIH and was until 2011, a member of its Council of Councils (the advisory board to the director).

For a decade he chaired the Department of Social Medicine at Harvard Medical School and from 1993–2000 he was Presley Professor in that department. He is currently professor of medical anthropology and psychiatry in the Department of Global Health and Social Medicine, Harvard Medical School. From 2004 through 2007, he chaired Harvard's Department of Anthropology (FAS), and since 2008 he has headed Harvard's Asia Center as Victor and William Fung Director. Since 2002 he has served as Esther and Sidney Rabb Professor of Anthropology. Kleinman is also a Harvard College Professor of Harvard University and was given the Distinguished Faculty Award by the Harvard Foundation for 2011.

Tami Kramer, PhD, is senior clinical research fellow at Imperial College London and Consultant Child & Adolescent Psychiatrist in CNWL NHS Trust. Her interests include primary care child and adolescent psychiatry, adolescent forensic psychiatry, and the internet and child and adolescent mental health.

Yoko Komine, Showa University, Karasuyama Hospital, Tokyo, Japan.

Grace M. Lilienthal, BS, is program assistant for the Research Program on Children and Global Adversity (RPCGA), directed by Dr. Theresa Betancourt at the Harvard School of Public Health. Prior to joining the

RPCGA team, she spent eight months in Rwanda working on development and post-genocide reconciliation efforts. She has served with organizations promoting the health and thriving of children and youth in China, El Salvador, Singapore, and in low-resource and school settings in the United States.

Lilienthal holds a BS in child development and political science from Vanderbilt University. Her interests include risk and resilience in populations facing multiple forms of adversity, mental health services research, and developmental psychology.

Ryan McBain, MSc, is a research associate at the FXB Center for Health and Human Rights and doctoral candidate in the Department of Global Health and Population at Harvard University. His research focus is on the development of evidence-based policies for vulnerable populations, including the provision of mental health services for young persons affected by war and complex trauma.

Marguerite Marlow, Department of Psychology at Stellenbosch University, South Africa.

Michel Maziade, MD, Centre de recherche de l'Institut universitaire en santé mentale de Québec, Canada, Département de Psychiatrie, Université Laval, Canada.

Kathleen Ries Merikangas, PhD, is senior investigator and chief of the Genetic Epidemiology Branch in the Intramural Research Program at the National Institute of Mental Health (NIMH). Dr. Merikangas received a bachelor's degree *summa cum laude* in experimental psychology and music from the University of Notre Dame. She received clinical training through an NIAAA-sponsored master's program and internship at the Western Psychiatric Institute and Clinic at the University of Pittsburgh School of Medicine, where she continued to conduct clinical research on the Affective Disorders Clinical Research Unit while she pursued a PhD in chronic disease epidemiology from the University of Pittsburgh School of Public Health. Through a Career Development Award from the NIMH, she completed postdoctoral training in population genetics/ genetic epidemiology at the Yale University School of Medicine, where she joined the faculty and ultimately became a professor of epidemiology and public health, psychiatry and psychology and the director of the Genetic Epidemiology Research Unit in the Department of Epidemiology and Public Health. She came to the NIH in 2002 as part of the development of the Mood Disorders Program in the Intramural Research Program at the NIMH.

Dr. Merikangas has authored more than 300 scientific publications and has presented lectures throughout the United States and in more than twenty countries. Her work has contributed to both methodology in epidemiology and genetics, including methods for studying causes of comorbidity and the development of the genome-wide association study approach to detect genes for complex diseases, and to substantive knowledge about comorbidity of mood disorders with substance use disorders in general population samples as well as in African Americans and migrant and non-migrant Puerto Rican families. Dr. Merikangas has also devoted substantial effort to training activities including mentorship of individuals and directing formal training programs in genetic epidemiology at both Yale and at the NIH. The two major areas of her research in the Intramural Program at the NIMH are population based studies of mental and physical disorders including the first study of mental disorders in a nationally representative sample of youth in the United States, and multigenerational family studies designed to identify the core features and biomarkers of genetic and environmental factors underlying the familial transmission of bipolar spectrum disorders and co-transmission of mood and anxiety disorders and migraine.

Marie-Rose Moro, MD, PhD, is professor of child and adolescent psychiatry, University Paris Descartes, and chief of the Department of Medicine and Adolescent Psychiatry, Cochin Hospital, INSERM Unit 669, Paris, France.

Elizabeth Newnham, MPsych, PhD, is assistant professor at The University of Western Australia and a research fellow at the FXB Center for Health and Human Rights at Harvard School of Public Health. Her research focuses on mental health outcomes and intervention for populations living in disaster, post-conflict and adverse environments. Dr. Newnham received her PhD and masters in clinical psychology from The University of Western Australia and holds a National Health and Medical Research Council of Australia Sidney Sax Fellowship, which supports her work.

Thomas Paccalet, PhD, Centre de recherche de l'Institut universitaire en santé mentale de Québec, Canada.

Rahmethnissah Radjack, MD, is child and adolescent psychiatrist in the Department of Medicine and Adolescent Psychiatry, Cochin Hospital, and a researcher at INSERM Unit 669, Paris.

Jean-Philippe Raynaud, MD, is professor of child and adolescent psychiatry and head of department at Toulouse University Hospital (Centre

Hospitalier Universitaire de Toulouse, France), member of the French National Institute of Health and Medical Research (INSERM UMR 1027), president of the Scientific Committee of French Society for Child and Adolescent Psychiatry (SFPEADA), and vice president of IACAPAP (International Society for Child and Adolescent Psychiatry and Allied Professions).

Jordan Sibeoni, MD, is child and adolescent psychiatrist in the Department of Medicine and Adolescent Psychiatry, Cochin Hospital, and a researcher at INSERM Unit 669, Paris.

Koen Stolk is in psychiatric training in The Hague and Leiden, in the Netherlands.

Mark Tomlinson is a professor in the Department of Psychology at Stellenbosch University, South Africa. His scholarly work has involved a diverse range of topics that have in common an interest in factors that contribute to compromised maternal health, to understanding infant and child development in contexts of high adversity and how to develop community-based intervention programs. He has a particular interest in understanding infant and child development in the context of caregiver mental illness. He has published over one hundred papers in peer-reviewed journals, edited two books, and published numerous chapters.

John Weisz, PhD, is professor in the psychology department in the Harvard University Faculty of Arts and Sciences, and also in Harvard Medical School. His research involves development and testing of interventions for child mental health problems, encompassing depression, anxiety, and disruptive conduct. He and his colleagues in the Harvard Lab for Youth Mental Health also conduct meta-analyses, characterizing and critiquing the evidence base in youth psychotherapy.

Dr. James Woollard is specialist registrar in child and adolescent mental health in London, UK, and has a research interest in applying technology to mental health care and the effects of the internet and social media on the mental health of young people.

Hideki Yokoi, Showa University, Karasuyama Hospital, Tokyo, Japan.